Khaoula Rekik
Mariem Zayet
Mounir Ben Jemaa

Urinary tract infection in the elderly

Khaoula Rekik
Mariem Zayet
Mounir Ben Jemaa

Urinary tract infection in the elderly

Special features

ScienciaScripts

Imprint

Any brand names and product names mentioned in this book are subject to trademark, brand or patent protection and are trademarks or registered trademarks of their respective holders. The use of brand names, product names, common names, trade names, product descriptions etc. even without a particular marking in this work is in no way to be construed to mean that such names may be regarded as unrestricted in respect of trademark and brand protection legislation and could thus be used by anyone.

Cover image: www.ingimage.com

This book is a translation from the original published under ISBN 978-620-6-72299-1.

Publisher:
Sciencia Scripts
is a trademark of
Dodo Books Indian Ocean Ltd. and OmniScriptum S.R.L publishing group

120 High Road, East Finchley, London, N2 9ED, United Kingdom
Str. Armeneasca 28/1, office 1, Chisinau MD-2012, Republic of Moldova, Europe
Printed at: see last page
ISBN: 978-620-8-14133-2

SUMMARY

INTRODUCTION

Urinary tract infection (UTI) in the elderly is a major public health problem due to its high frequency and potentially serious consequences (1) . With increasing life expectancy, the proportion of elderly people in the general population continues to grow, thus increasing the number of patients at risk of UTIs (2) . The clinical and therapeutic particularities of UTI in the elderly are multiple and complex, justifying particular attention both in diagnosis and therapeutic management (1) .

Urinary tract infections are defined by the presence of pathogenic germs in the urine, leading to inflammation of the urinary tract. In the elderly, the clinical presentation of UTI often differs from that observed in young adults. Classic symptoms such as dysuria, urinary urgency, and low back pain may be absent or less pronounced. Atypical manifestations such as cognitive impairment, impaired general condition, unexplained falls, or new or worsening urinary incontinence may reveal UTI. These clinical features make the diagnosis of UTI more difficult in the elderly, requiring increased vigilance on the part of healthcare professionals (3) .

Several factors predispose older adults to UTIs. Age-related physiological changes, such as decreased immune function, reduced mobility, and the presence of comorbidities, increase the risk of developing UTIs. In addition, frequent use of medical devices such as urinary catheters, surgical procedures, and polypharmacy also increase this risk. Anatomical changes, such as prostatic hypertrophy in men and postmenopausal urogenital atrophy in women, also contribute to increased susceptibility to UTIs (3) .

The treatment of urinary tract infections in the elderly poses specific challenges. Therapeutic choices must take into account the often impaired renal function, the high risk of adverse drug reactions and the frequent presence of multidrug-resistant bacteria. The management of UTIs in the elderly therefore requires an individualized approach, integrating precise clinical and microbiological criteria. The duration of treatment, the route of administration of antibiotics, as well as the need for close monitoring are crucial elements in the management of these patients (1) .

Prevention of UTIs in older adults is of particular importance. Preventive measures, such as adequate hydration, treatment of underlying conditions, and education of patients and caregivers on good urinary hygiene practices, can reduce the incidence of UTIs. In addition, rational use of antibiotics is essential to limit the emergence of bacterial resistance (3) .

As part of the study of this pathology in elderly patients and to better support these particularities, we conducted a study with the following objectives:

- ❖ To study the epidemiological, clinical and paraclinical characteristics of urinary tract infection in the elderly.
- ❖ Detail the therapeutic management of this clinical entity.

PATIENTS AND METHODS

1. TYPE OF STUDY

We conducted a retrospective descriptive study of the files of elderly patients followed in the infectious diseases department of the Hédi Chaker University Hospital in Sfax between January 2010 and December 2022 for a urinary tract infection.

2. DEFINITION OF THE STUDY POPULATION

2.1. Inclusion criteria

We included in our study all patients aged over 65 years followed during our study period and treated for a urinary tract infection.

The diagnosis of this infection was made in any patient with clinical symptoms suggestive of urinary tract infection (burning on urination, pollakiuria, dysuria, polyuria, etc.) with or without an abnormality in the examination of the urinary tract (painful lumbar shock, painful digital rectal examination in men, etc.) with a pathological cytobacteriological examination of the urine (ECBU) defined by pathological leukocyturia ($> 10,000$ EB/ml or $10/mm^3$) and a positive culture for a pathogenic germ with a germ density $\geq 10^3$ CFU/ml in men and in women a density $\geq 10^3$ CFU/ml for *Escherichia coli* and *Staphylococcus saprophyticus* and $\geq 10^4$ CFU/ml for other bacteria (enterobacteria other than *E. coli* , enterococci…).

For healthcare-associated infections, in the absence of an endo-urinary device, it is strongly recommended to use the same thresholds as for community-acquired infections. In the presence of an endo-urinary device, leukocyturia is not predictive of the presence or absence of a urinary tract infection and does not enter into the criteria defining catheter-related urinary tract infection. It is strongly recommended to use the threshold of 10^5 CFU/ml for bacteriuria.

2.2. Non-inclusion criteria

We did not include patients whose age was less than 65 years, or who had records with missing or inconclusive data.

We did not include patients with a urine culture positive for more than one bacteria or yeast.

3. DEFINITIONS USED

3.1. Community-acquired urinary tract infection

Community-acquired urinary tract infection (CUTI) is an infection that develops within 48 hours of admission to hospital or in a patient from home (4) .

3.2. Nosocomial urinary tract infection

An infection is said to be nosocomial if it is absent when the patient is admitted to hospital and develops at least 48 hours after admission or a period longer than the incubation period.

3.3. Multi-resistant bacteria

A bacterium is said to be multiresistant if it is resistant to 3 families of antibiotics to which it is usually sensitive.

3.4. Ultra-resistant bacteria

A bacterium is said to be ultraresistant if it has acquired resistance to more than 1 molecule belonging to all ATB families except 1 or 2.

3.5. Types of urinary tract infections

⁜ Asymptomatic bacteriuria

Asymptomatic bacteriuria (ASB) is the presence of an infectious agent in the urine without associated clinical manifestations, regardless of the level of leukocyturia (4) .

In practice, this is a situation where treatment is only indicated in two situations:

❖ Pregnant woman from 4 months of pregnancy with bacteriuria $\geq 10^5$ CFU/mL

❖ Before an intervention on the urinary tract.

Cystitis

It is the infection of the bladder wall. It manifests itself by burning during urination, pollakiuria, dysuria, urgency, hypogastric pain and sometimes urinary incontinence. Without fever or lumbar pain. The presence of macroscopic hematuria is usual. Bacteriological confirmation is done by a urine dipstick and/or a pathological urine culture (4) .

Acute pyelonephritis (APN):

PNA is suspected in the event of sudden onset of signs of cystitis with signs of damage to the renal parenchyma and the renal collecting system (4) :

❖ Fever > 38.5°C, chills, general malaise

❖ Lower back pain, or costovertebral pain, most often unilateral, which can radiate under the ribs or go down towards the pubis, suggesting renal colic

❖ Digestive disorders (nausea, vomiting, diarrhea, bloating).

❖ Sometimes the picture is incomplete with behavioral disorder or sliding syndrome in the elderly.

Male urinary tract infection (MUI)

Frequently represented by acute prostatitis: This pathological entity is based on symptoms: infectious syndrome (fever, chills, general malaise) associated with urinary signs (pollakiuria, nocturia, urgency, dysuria and burning urination, etc.) (4) .

These signs may be associated with bladder retention with pelvic, perineal, ureteral pain with clinical examination looking for (4) :

❖ A bladder globe

❖ On rectal examination:

➢ A painful prostate,

➢ A fluctuating prostate suggesting an abscess.

❖ Signs of associated epididymitis or epididymo- orchitis .

Simple urinary tract infections

These are infections without risk factors for complications. They include simple cystitis and simple pyelonephritis in young women without risk factors for complications (4) .

Urinary tract infections known as risk of complications

They occur in patients with at least one complication risk factor (CRF) that can make the infection more complex (4) .

These risk factors for complications are (4) :

❖ Any organic or functional abnormality of the urinary tract whatsoever (bladder residue, reflux, lithiasis, tumor, recent act, etc.)

❖ Male gender, due to the frequency of underlying anatomical or functional abnormalities

❖ Pregnancy

❖ Elderly subject: patient aged 65 to 75 years with $\geq$ 3 fragility criteria (Fried criteria) (6) ,

❖ Age over 75 years.

❖ Severe immunosuppression

❖ Severe chronic renal failure (clearance $<$ 30ml/min)

❖ Namely, Fried's criteria are (6) :

➢ Unintentional weight loss in the past year

➢ Slow walking speed

➢ Low endurance

➢ Weakness/Fatigue

➢ Reduced physical activity

In our series, we considered all patients over 65 years of age as elderly subjects regardless of Fried's criteria.

Recurrent urinary tract infection

Defined by the occurrence of 4 episodes of urinary tract infection during 12 months or 3 episodes during 6 months (4) .

Serious urinary tract infection:

Urinary tract infection is considered serious if it is associated with (4) :

- Sepsis
- A state of septic shock
- An indication for a urological drainage procedure (surgical or by interventional radiology)

3.6. Systemic inflammatory response syndrome (SIRS)

SIRS is defined by the presence of two criteria out of a set of four following clinical -biological criteria:

- Temperature > 38.3°C or < 36°C
- Heart rate > 90 bpm/min
- Respiratory rate or $PaCO_2$ > 20/min or $PaCO_2$ < 32 mmHg
- Leukocytosis >12000 or <4000/mm3 [or] > 10% of immature forms.

3.7. Sepsis

Sepsis is defined as organ dysfunction secondary to an inappropriate host response to a documented or suspected infection (7) .

Organ dysfunction is defined by a " Sequential " score Organ Failure Assessment (SOFA) $\geq$ 2 or an increase in score of $\geq$ 2 points if organ dysfunction was present before infection (7) .

The quick SOFA (qSOFA) is a simple scoring system that can be repeatedly assessed at the bedside. The qSOFA criteria are (at least 2 of the below) (7) :

- Respiratory rate $\geq$ 22/min

- ❖ Altered neurological status (GCS ≤ 13)
- ❖ Systolic blood pressure ≤ 100 mmHg .

Sepsis according to the old definition is the association of SIRS and a clinically or microbiologically documented infection.

3.8. Severe or serious sepsis

Sepsis is considered severe when it is associated with one or more of the following organ dysfunctions:

1. Higher functions:

Presence of encephalopathy or confusional syndrome, which can be confirmed by measuring Glasgow score <14.

2. Renal function:

- ❖ Oliguria < 0.5ml/kg for 3 hours
- ❖ Creatinine > 177 µmol/L (20 mg/L), or 50% elevation from baseline.

3. Respiratory function:

- ❖ Pa02 < 60 mmHg or SpO2 < 90% in room air (or under 02)
- ❖ Pa02/FiO2 < 300, or decrease in this ratio >20% in patients receiving mechanical ventilation.

4. Coagulation:

- ❖ Thrombocytopenia < 100,000/mm3 ^{or} TP < 50%, or drop > 30% in platelet count or TP during 2 successive samples
- ❖ Disseminated intravascular coagulation score (International Society on Thrombosis and Haemostasis) > 4.

5. Liver function: Hyperbilirubinemia > 34 mmol /L

Circulatory function :

- ❖ Systolic blood pressure < 90 mmHg (or 40 mmHg decrease from baseline) or mean < 70 mmHg
- ❖ hyperlactatemia > 2 mmol /L
- ❖ In patients under hemodynamic monitoring, appearance of a hyperdynamic state (increase in cardiac index > 3.5 L/min.m ^{2}).

3.9. Septic shock state

Septic shock is defined by the presence of sepsis with persistent hypotension, despite vascular filling requiring the use of vasopressor amines, in order to maintain a mean arterial pressure (MAP) $\geq$ 65 mmHg and hyperlactatemia $\geq$ 2 mmol /l (7) .

According to the old definition, septic shock was defined as the persistence of hypotension despite adequate vascular filling during severe sepsis with the need for the introduction of vasopressors.

3.10. Acute renal failure

AKI is defined by a sudden and rapid decrease in glomerular filtration rate (GFR) leading to nitrogen retention, and hydroelectrolytic and acid- base disorders that can be life-threatening in the short term and renal prognosis in the long term (8) .

The diagnosis of acute character is based on the international recommendations KDIGO (Kidney Disease Improving Global Outcomes) from 2012 which are based on an increase in serum creatinine and/or a decrease in diuresis (8) .

3. 11. Chronic renal failure and chronic kidney disease

Chronic kidney disease (CKD) is defined by (9) :

- ❖ **1)** Presence of chronic renal failure (CRF) defined by a decrease in the estimated glomerular filtration rate (eGFR) < 60 mL /min/1.73 m² (CKD-EPI formula).
- ❖ **2)** Or presence of at least one marker of renal damage persisting for more than 3 months:
  - ➢ Albuminuria or proteinuria
  - ➢ Hematuria > 10/mm³ (excluding urological causes)
  - ➢ Leukocyturia > 10/mm³ (in the absence of infection)

➢ Morphological abnormality on renal ultrasound

➢ Size asymmetry, bumpy contours, small kidneys or large polycystic kidneys, nephrocalcinosis, cyst.

3.12. Evolutionary data

3.12.1. Favorable evolution

This is the improvement of clinical signs after the start of antibiotic treatment with complete disappearance of clinical signs.

3.12.2. Unfavorable development

3.12.2.1. Relapse

This is the resumption of clinical symptoms with isolation of the same germ at the beginning of the convalescence period or in the first month following the initial episode. It is due either to treatment failure or to poor adherence to the proposed therapy.

3.12.2.2. Repeat offense

This is the reappearance of clinical signs with isolation of the same germ after one month of stopping treatment for the initial infection.

3. 12.2.3. Persistence

It is the persistence of the same germ initially isolated in the urine, with or without improvement of clinical signs, at the end of a curative and complete treatment.

3.12.2.4. Reinfection

This is the resumption of clinical signs with isolation of a germ different from that of the initial infection after stopping treatment and clinical and microbiological recovery.

4. METHODS

Data collection was carried out from files archived in the department.

Data collection was carried out on a pre-established form including:

- **Epidemiological data**

  - ❖ Age, gender.
  - ❖ Medical and surgical history and risk factors.

- **Clinical data**

  - ❖ Time to diagnosis (defined as the average time between the onset of symptoms and the diagnosis of UI).
  - ❖ Functional signs, signs of severity.

- **Biological data (Annex 2)**

  - ❖ Blood count and formula (CBC) (looking for anemia, inflammatory syndrome, neutrophil-predominant leukocytosis or leukopenia; thrombocytosis; thrombocytopenia)
  - ❖ Sedimentation rate (SSR)
  - ❖ C-reactive protein (CRP)
  - ❖ Blood sugar looking for diabetes or hypoglycemia;
  - ❖ Estimation of GFR in search of renal failure;

- **Bacteriological diagnosis**

  - ❖ Blood culture to isolate the germ(s) in the event of septicemia.
  - ❖ Cytobacteriological examination of urine (ECBU) to search for pathogenic germs, leukocyturia and microscopic hematuria.
  - ❖ Antibiogram looking for antibiotics active on the germ in question.

- **Radiological data**

  - ❖ Ultrasound of the kidneys and urinary tract,
  - ❖ CT scan (urinary tract abnormality, kidney obstruction or pain).

- **Therapeutic data**

  - ❖ Antibiotics used (dosage, route of administration and duration of treatment)
  - ❖ Interventional radiology (drainage and puncture) and surgery.

⊥ Scalable data

❖ Favorable: apyrexia and disappearance of other symptoms.

❖ Unfavorable development:

➢ Relapse

➢ Recidivism

➢ Reinfection

➢ Persistence

➢ Death.

5. STATISTICAL STUDY

Data entry and statistical analysis of the different variables were done using SPSS 27 software.

We expressed qualitative variables as frequencies (percentages) and quantitative variables as means ± standard deviation (SD) after checking the normality of the distribution, or as median and interquartile range if the normality of the distribution was not verified.

The Kolmogorov-Smirnov test (number > 50 individuals) was used to check the normality of the distribution of quantitative variables.

RESULTS

1. EPIDEMIOLOGY

During the 13 years of the study, we collected 382 cases of patients aged over 65 who were followed for a urinary tract infection.

The mean annual frequency was 29.4 cases/year with extremes of 19 to 45 cases/year (Figure 1).

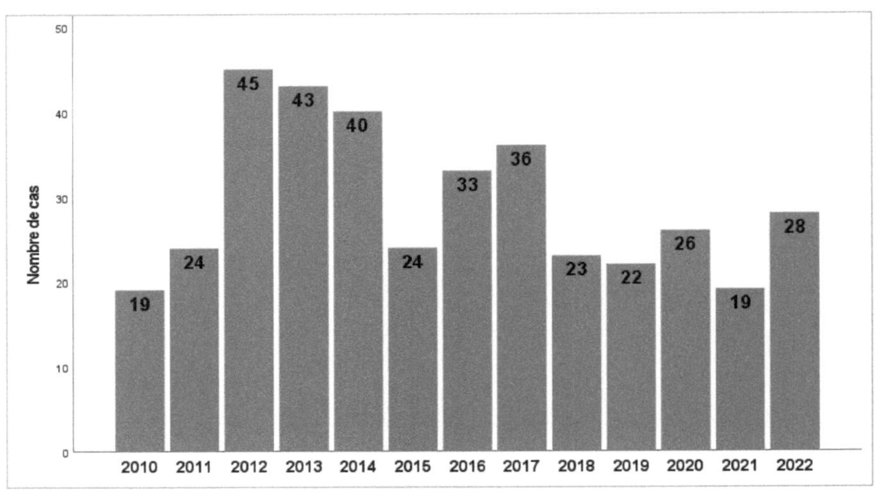

Figure 1: Annual distribution of patients

The average monthly frequency was 2.4 cases/month with a maximum of 10 cases/month.

The seasonal distribution of patients showed a summer predominance (30.9%) (Figure 2).

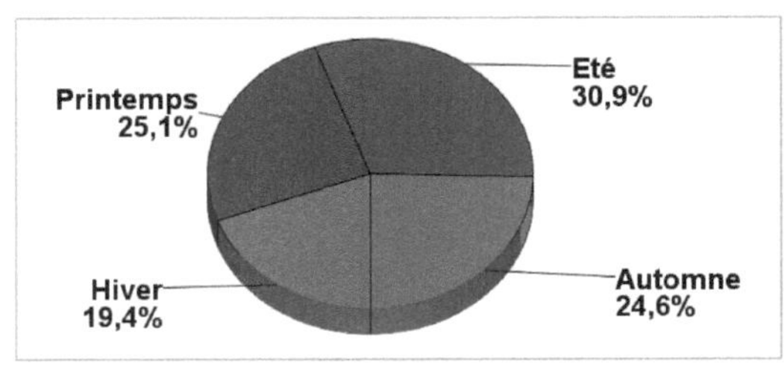

Figure 2: Seasonal distribution of urinary tract infection

2. SOCIODEMOGRAPHIC CHARACTERISTICS OF THE STUDY POPULATION

2.1. Age

The mean age of our patients was 75.6±6.5 years with extremes ranging from 65 to 97 years.

The most affected age group was adults aged between 65 and 80 years (295 cases: 77.2%) (Figure 3).

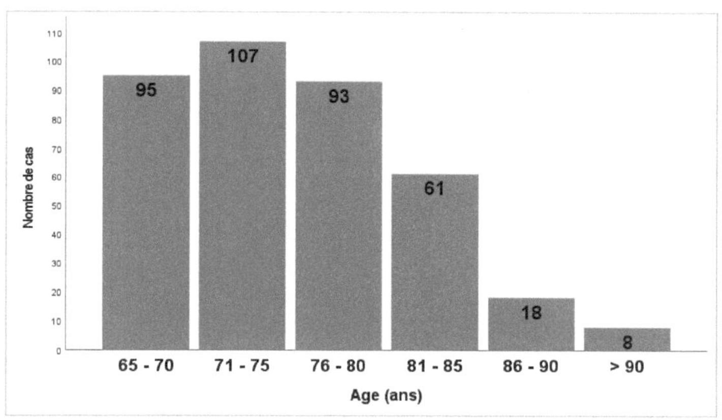

Figure 3: Distribution of patients by age

2.2. Sex

We noted a female predominance (52.6%) with a male/female sex ratio equal to 0.9 (Figure 4).

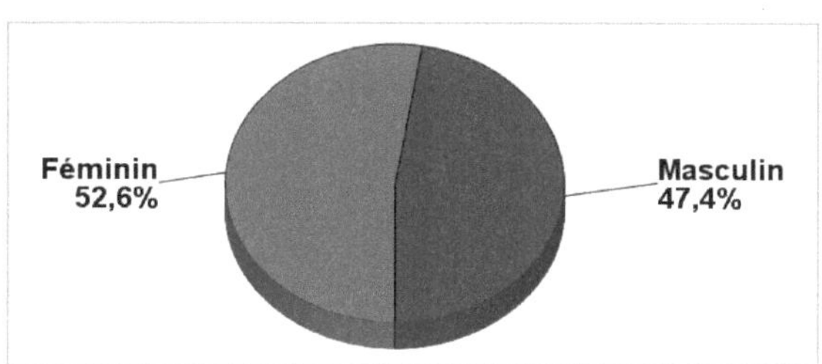

Figure 4: Distribution of patients by gender

3. PERSONAL BACKGROUND

Personal history was noted in 312 cases (81.7%).

3.1. Medical history

Medical history was dominated by diabetes (50.5%), high blood pressure (45%) and stroke (9.4%) (Table I). In addition, one hundred and one patients had a history of previous hospitalization (26.4%).

Table I: Frequency of medical history

Medical history	Number of patients	Percentage (%)
Diabetes	193	50.5
High blood pressure	172	45
Stroke	36	9.4
Coronary artery disease	34	8.9
Complete arrhythmia due to atrial fibrillation	16	4.2
Heart failure	6	1.5
Acute pulmonary edema	2	0.5
Pacemaker	2	0.5
Pericarditis	2	0.5

3.2. Nephro -urological history

most common nephro -urological antecedents were acute pyelonephritis (23.8%) and urinary stones (14.7%) (Table II).

Table II: Frequency of nephro -urological history

Nephro -urological history	Number of patients	Percentage (%)
Acute pyelonephritis	91	23.8
Urinary lithiasis	56	14.7
Benign prostatic hyperplasia	49	12.8
Acute pyelonephritis due to multi-drug resistant bacteria	37	9.7
Chronic renal failure	37	9.7
Recurrent urinary tract infections	34	8.9
Renal colic	21	5.5
Neurological bladder	21	5.5
Urinary tumor	17	4.5
Urinary malformation	7	1.8
Indwelling urinary catheter	6	1.6
Urinary tuberculosis	2	0.5

4. CLINICAL DATA

4.1. Origin of urinary tract infection

The 382 Confirmed urinary tract infections were classified as community-acquired in 351 cases (91.9%) and nosocomial in 31 cases (8.1%) (Figure 5).

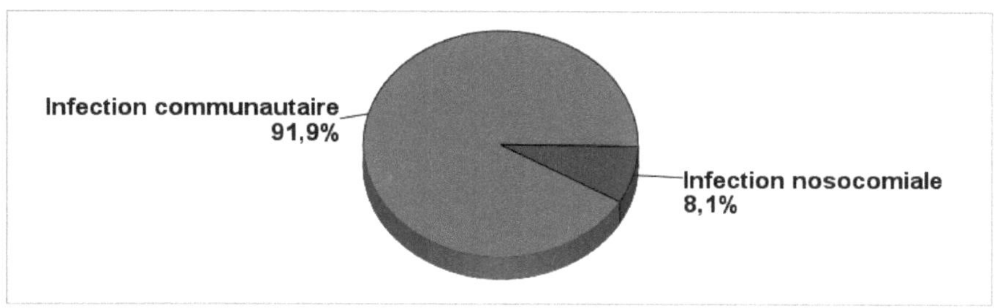

Figure 5: Distribution of patients according to the type of urinary tract infection

For nosocomial origin, the infection was mainly following a stay in a hospital department (64.5%) (Figure 6).

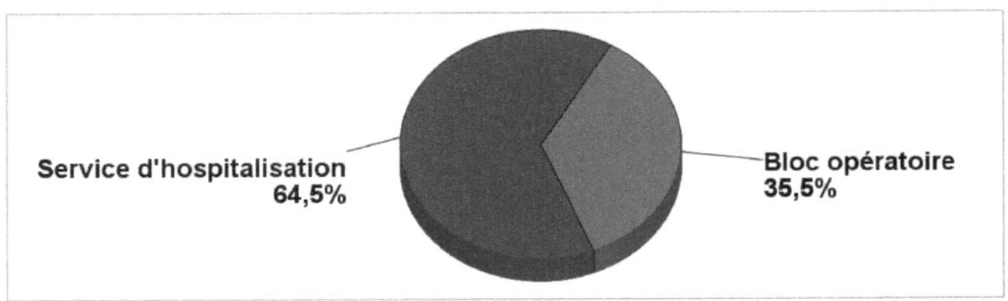

Figure 6: Distribution of patients according to the origin of the nosocomial urinary tract infection

4.2. Functional signs

Suprapubic pain was the most common functional sign (79.6%) (Table III).

Table III: Distribution of patients according to functional signs

Clinical forms	Number of patients	Percentage (%)
Suprapubic pain	304	79.6
Lower back pain	299	78.3
Pollakiuria	255	66.8
Hematuria	181	47.4
Urinary incontinence	127	33.2
Urgenturia	103	27
Behavioral disorders	69	18.1
Confusion	39	10.2
Delirium	25	6.5

4.3. Physical examination

The mean temperature was $37.9 \pm 0.9°C$ with extremes ranging from 36 to 41°C. Fever was found in 196 patients (51.3%).

Systolic blood pressure had a mean of 123 ± 20 mmHg (range 70 to 180 mmHg) and diastolic blood pressure had a mean of 68 ± 11 mmHg (range 30 to 110 mmHg).

4.4 . Clinical forms

Acute pyelonephritis was the most observed clinical form (84.8%) (Table IV).

Table IV: Distribution of patients according to clinical forms .

Clinical forms	Number of patients	Percentage (%)
Acute pyelonephritis	324	84.8
Cystitis	24	6.3
Prostatitis	19	5
Orchid - epididymitis	7	1.8
Kidney abscess	6	1.6
Acute emphysematous pyelonephritis	1	0.3
Prostatic abscess	1	0.3

4.5. Signs of severity

Systemic inflammatory response syndrome (SIRS) was the most common sign of severity (47.4%) (Table V).

The qSOFA was greater than or equal to two in 90 cases (25.9%).

Table V: Distribution of patients according to the severity of the clinical form

Clinical forms	Number of patients	Percentage (%)
Systemic inflammatory response syndrome	181	47.4
qSOFA ≥ 2	90	25.9
Sepsis	79	20.7
Severe sepsis	14	3.7
Septic shock state	6	1.6

4.6. Hospitalization

Among our patients, 310 (81.2%) were hospitalized with an average duration of 8 days (from 1 day to 2 months).

5. PARACLINICAL DATA

5.1. Biological data

Hyperleukocytosis ($\geq$ 10000/mm3 $^)$ was noted in 226 patients (59.1%). Leukopenia (< 4000/mm3 $^)$ was noted in 35 patients (9.1%).

CRP was negative ($\leq$ 10 mg/l) in 41 patients (10.7%), positive (> 10 mg/l) in 309 patients (80.9%).

Creatinine was > 120 µmol /L in 179 patients (46.8%) (Table VI).

Table VI: Biological data of patients

Biological data	Average	Standard deviation	Minimum	Maximum
C-reactive protein (mg/l)	140	102	6	416
Blood count and formula				
White blood cells (WB/mm³)	13,524	11,660	630	194,000
Polynuclear neutrophils (EB/mm³)	10,521	6,406	1090	35 320
Lymphocytes (EB/mm³)	1,574	1 102	240	9,200
Platelets (elements/mm³)	238,974	105,066	76,000	722,000
Kidney function				
Creatinine level (µmol /l)	152	109	32	761
Other settings				
Natremia (mmol /l)	134	5	120	158
Kaliemia (mmol /l)	4	0.6	2.4	5.3
Aspartate aminotransferase (IU/l)	29	28	4	201
Alanine aminotransferase (IU/l)	24	21	3	163

5.2. Microbiology

5.2.1. Macroscopic appearance of urine

Macroscopically, urine was cloudy in 96.1% of cases (Table VII).

Table VII: Distribution of patients according to the macroscopic appearance of urine

Macroscopic appearance of urine	Number of patients	Percentage (%)
Cloudy appearance	367	96.1
Clear appearance	13	3.4
Hematic aspect	2	0.5

5.2.2. Urine cytology

Pathological leukocyturia was present in 358 patients (93.7%) and microscopic hematuria was found in 18 cases (4.7%).

5.2.3. Urine culture

Escherichia *coli* was the most isolated germ (62.8%) (Table VIII) .

Table VIII: Distribution of patients according to germs isolated in urine .

Family	Germs isolated in urine	Number of cases	Percentage (%)
Enterobacteria *N = 349 (91.2%)*	*Escherichia coli*	240	62.8
	Klebsiella pneumoniae	78	20.3
	Proteus mirabilis	10	2.6
	Other enterobacteria*	21	5.5
Gram positive cocci *N = 18 (4.8%)*	*Staphylococcus aureus*	5	1.3
	Streptococcus B	3	0.8
	Enterococcus faecalis	9	2.4
	Enterococcus faecium	1	0.3
Gram-negative bacilli *Non-fermentative* *N = 15 (4%)*	*Pseudomonas aeruginosa*	13	3.4
	Burkholderia cepacia	1	0.3
	Acinetobacter	1	0.3
Total		**382**	**100**

Enterobacter cloacae , Morganella morgani , Serratia marcescens , Providencia stuarti , Klebsiella oxytoca

The most isolated germ in cases of nosocomial UTI was *Klebsiella pneumoniae* (n=12; 38.7%) (Table IX).

Table IX: Distribution of germs isolated in urine according to the type of infection

Germs isolated in urine	Community infection (n =351)		Nosocomial infection (n =31)	
	N	Percentage (%)	N	Percentage (%)
Enterobacteria	323	83.5	26	87.1
Escherichia coli	230	62.7	10	32.3
Klebsiella pneumoniae	66	18.8	12	38.7
Proteus mirabilis	9	2.6	1	3.2
Other enterobacteria	18	5.2	3	9.6
Gram positive cocci	16	4.3	2	6.4
Staphylococcus aureus	4	1.1	1	3.2
Streptococcus B	2	0.6	1	3.2
Enterococcus faecalis	9	2.6	0	0
Enterococcus faecium	1	0.3	0	0
Non-fermenting Gram-negative bacilli	12	3.1	3	9.7
Pseudomonas aeruginosa	11	3.1	2	6.5
Burkholderia cepacia	0	0	1	3.2
tobacter	1	0.3	0	0

5.2.4. Urine antibiogram

5.2.4.1. Sensitivity profile of enterobacteria strains

For the Enterobacteriaceae strains tested, we found a susceptibility to imipenem of 94.6%, to amikacin of 92%, to amoxicillin of 15.5% and to amoxicillin/clavulanic acid of 44% (Table X).

Table X: Sensitivity of Enterobacteria to antibiotics.

	Antibiotics	Enterobacteria sensitivity (%)
Beta-lactams	Amoxicillin	15.5
	Amoxicillin-Clavulanic Acid	44
	Ceftriaxone	66.4
	Cefoxitin	74
	Ceftazidime	66.9
	Imipenem	94.6
Aminoglycosides	Gentamicin	69
	Amikacin	92
Phenicolaceae	Chloramphenicol	77.3
Quinolones	Nalidixic Acid	49.1
	Ciprofloxacin	49.8
Polymyxins	Colistin	86.9
Furans	Nitrofurantoin	82.6
Fosfomycin	Fosfomycin	90.2

5.2.4.2. Sensitivity profile of *Escherichia coli strains*

Escherichia coli strains tested, we found a susceptibility to colistin of 98.5%, to imipenem of 97.8%, to amoxicillin of 24% and to amoxicillin/clavulanic acid of 50% (Table XI).

Table XI: Sensitivity of *Escherichia coli strains* to antibiotics .

Antibiotics		*Escherichia coli* sensitivity (%)
Beta-lactams	Amoxicillin	24
	Amoxicillin-Clavulanic Acid	50
	Ceftriaxone	76.3
	Cefoxitin	84
	Ceftazidime	75
	Imipenem	97.8
Aminoglycosides	Gentamicin	74.9
	Amikacin	93.2
Phenicolaceae	Chloramphenicol	86.5
Quinolones	Nalidixic Acid	55
	Ciprofloxacin	55.9
Polymyxins	Colistin	98.5
Furans	Nitrofurantoin	97.5
Fosfomycin	Fosfomycin	96.6

5.2.4.3. Susceptibility profile of *Klebsiella pneumoniae strains*

Klebsiella pneumoniae strains tested, we found a susceptibility to colistin of 94.1%, to amikacin of 84.1%, and to amoxicillin/clavulanic acid of 28.9% (Table XII).

Table I*Klebsiella pneumoniae* strains to antibiotics

	Antibiotics	*Klebsiella pneumoniae* susceptibility (%)
Beta-lactams	Amoxicillin-Clavulanic Acid	28.9
	Ceftriaxone	38.2
	Cefoxitin	51.4
	Ceftazidime	36.8
	Imipenem	81.6
Aminoglycosides	Gentamicin	48.5
	Amikacin	84.1
Phenicolaceae	Chloramphenicol	63
Quinolones	Nalidixic Acid	31
	Ciprofloxacin	28.9
Polymyxins	Colistin	94.1
Furans	Nitrofurantoin	57.6
Fosfomycin	Fosfomycin	75.3

Compared to community infections, nosocomial infections were significantly due to multiresistant germs (77.4%) (Table XIV).

Table XIII: Distribution of multidrug-resistant bacteria according to the type of urinary tract infection.

Germs isolated in urine	Community infection (n =351)		Nosocomial infection (n =31)	
	N	Percentage (%)	N	Percentage (%)
Multi-resistant	166	47.3	25	80.6
Ultra-resistant	18	5.2	5	16.2
Sensitive	167	47.5	1	3.2
Total	351	100	31	100

5.2.5. Blood culture

Blood cultures were performed in 195 cases (51%). They were positive in 63 patients (16.5%). Escherichia *coli was* the most isolated germ (n=34; 53.9%) followed by *Klebsiella pneumoniae* (n=12; 19%).

6. IMAGING

6.1. Ultrasound

Ultrasound was performed in 308 patients (80.6%). It was without abnormalities in 83 cases (21.8%).

The most common renal abnormalities were simple renal cysts (20.8%) and chronic renal disease kidneys (15.9%) (Table IV).

Table XIV: Renal abnormalities found on ultrasound .

Kidney abnormalities	Number of patients	Percentage (%)
Simple renal cysts	64	20.8
Chronic kidney disease	49	15.9
Hydronephrosis without detectable obstruction	49	15.9
Kidney stones	48	15.6
Pyelic thickening	10	3.2
Kidney abscess	6	1.9
Single kidney	1	0.3
Polycystic kidney disease	1	0.3

Prostatic hypertrophy was noted in 29 patients (9.4%) (Table XV).

Table XV: Abnormalities found on ultrasound .

Ultrasound abnormalities	Number of patients	Percentage (%)
Prostate hypertrophy	29	9.4
Metabolic overload liver	25	8.1
Simple gallbladder lithiasis	10	3.2
Bladder lithiasis	5	1.6
Orchid - epididymitis	3	0.9
Epididymitis	2	0.6
Bladder thickening covering the 2 ureteral meatuses and dilation upstream	1	0.3
Prostatic abscess	1	0.3

6.2 . Abdominal CT scan

Abdominal CT scan, performed in 69 patients (18%), showed essentially pyelocaliceal dilatation in the vicinity of a stone in 20 cases (28.4%).

Other anomalies noted were:

* Aspect in favor of obstructive PNA in 9 cases (13%)
* Bilateral pyelocaliceal junction syndrome, vesicoureteral reflux and simple renal cysts in 5 cases (7.2%) each
* Renal abscess in 6 cases (8.7%)
* Emphysematous PNA in 1 case (1.4%)
* Obstructive ureteral stone with multiple renal stones including one at the obstructive pyelocaliceal junction in 1 case (1.4%),
* Low-abundance retroperitoneal effusion at the level of the right renal compartment in 1 case (1.4%).

7. THERAPEUTIC DATA OF THE POPULATION

7.1. Medical treatment

7.1.1. Empirical antibiotic therapy before hospitalization

In our population, 94 patients (24.6%) received probabilistic antibiotic therapy before hospitalization. Third-generation cephalosporins were the most prescribed molecules in 35 cases (37.2%) followed by fluoroquinolones in 24 cases (25.5%) (Figure 7).

For cases of cystitis, treatment was based on fosfomycin trometamol in all cases.

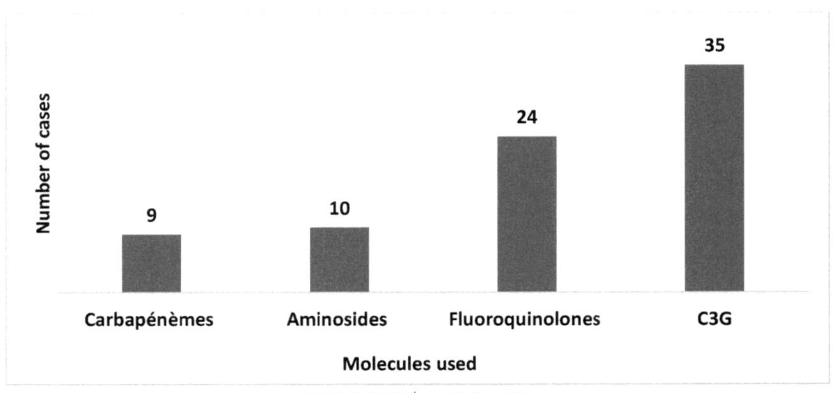

*C3G: 3rd generation cephalosporins

Figure 7: Empirical antibiotic therapy prescribed before hospitalization.

7.1.2. Empirical antibiotic therapy on admission

Empirical antibiotic therapy was prescribed in all patients (100%) on the day of admission. Third-generation cephalosporins were the most prescribed molecules in 214 cases (56%) followed by fluoroquinolones in 125 cases (32.7%).

Figure 8 summarizes the main molecules empirically prescribed for our study population.

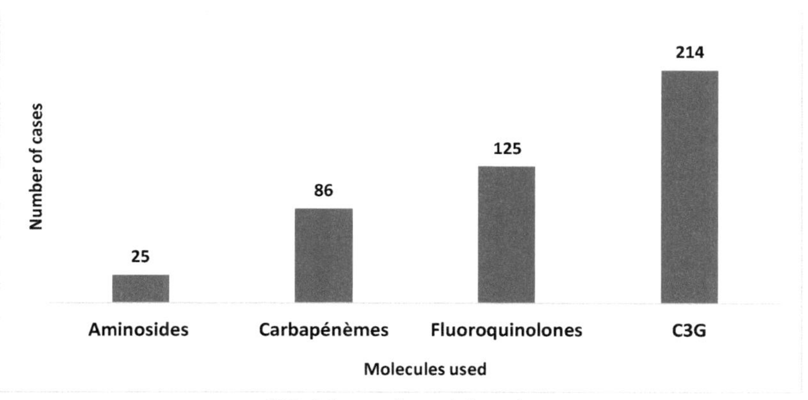

C3G: 3rd generation cephalosporins

Figure 8: Antibiotic therapy prescribed on the day of admission

Furthermore, empirical antibiotic therapy varied according to the clinical picture. The main molecules used according to the clinical form are presented in Table XVI.

Table XVI: Antibiotic therapy according to clinical form.

Clinical form	Total number of cases	Empirical antibiotic therapy	Number of cases (%)
PNA	324	C3G Fluoroquinolones	195 (60.2) 45 (13.9)
IUM	27	Fluoroquinolones	16 (59.2)
Kidney abscess	6	C3G + fluoroquinolone Imipenem + fluoroquinolone	4 (66.6) 2 (33.4)

| Emphysematous PNA | 1 | C3G + fluoroquinolone + aminoglycoside | 1 (100) |

PNA: Acute pyelonephritis, IUM: male urinary tract infection, C3G: 3rd generation cephalosporins

7.1.3. Antibiotic therapy after documentation

Antibiotic treatment after bacteriological documentation was adapted to empirical antibiotic therapy in 334 cases (87.4%).

The main molecules used after bacteriological documentation are presented in Table XVII.

Table II: Main molecules of relay antibiotic therapy

Relay antibiotic therapy	Number of cases	Percentage (%)
Carbapenems	142	37.2
Fluoroquinolones	95	24.9
3rd generation cephalosporin	82	21.5
Trimethoprim + Sulfamethoxazole	45	11.7

7.1.4. Total duration of antibiotic therapy

The median duration of total antibiotic therapy was 14 ± 9 days with extremes [1-92 days].

Table XVIII shows the duration of antibiotic treatment according to the clinical form.

Table III: Duration of treatment according to clinical form.

Clinical form	Median duration of treatment
Acute pyelonephritis	10 ±2 days
Prostatitis	18±4 days
Kidney abscess	32 ± 3 days

Treatment of cystitis was one minute treatment in 40% of cases and 3 separate doses of fosfomycin trometamol in the remaining cases.

7.2. Surgical or interventional treatment

Surgical or interventional treatment was considered in 16 patients (4.2%). This consisted of drainage by double-J ureteral catheterization in 9 cases (2.4%) and radiological percutaneous renal drainage in 7 cases (1.8%).

8. EVOLUTION

8.1. Favorable evolution

A favorable evolution was noted in 289 patients (75.6%) and the mean time to apyrexia was 2.1 ± 1.9 days with extremes of 1 to 20 days.

8.1. Unfavorable developments

An unfavorable evolution was found in 81 patients (21.2%) (Table XIX). The mortality rate was 3.1% (n=12).

Table IV: Distribution of patients according to unfavorable evolution

Unfavorable evolution	Number of patients	Percentage (%)
Reinfection	38	9.9
Recidivism	18	4.7
Persistence	14	3.7
Relapse	11	2.9

DISCUSSION

1. EPIDEMIOLOGY OF URINARY TRACT INFECTION IN THE ELDERLY

The prevalence of urinary tract infection increases with age and depends on the place of residence. In the community setting, it ranks second after bronchopulmonary infections (3) .

It is the most commonly diagnosed infection in long-term care facility residents, accounting for more than one-third of all nursing home-associated infections (3,4). It is second only to respiratory infections in hospitalized patients and adults over 65 years of age living in the community (6,7).

As our population ages, the burden of UTIs in older adults is expected to increase, which may make improved diagnostic and preventive strategies necessary (1).

Although several estimates exist in the literature, it is difficult to accurately measure the incidence of UTIs in the elderly because the criteria used for diagnosis are not consistent in epidemiological studies. In addition, it is difficult to differentiate UTI from asymptomatic bacteriuria (ABB) and misclassification may occur (1).

1.1. Incidence of urinary tract infections in the elderly

The incidence of UTIs is higher in women than in men in all age groups. UTIs are common in young sexually active women with reported incidence rates ranging from 0.5 to 0.7 per person-year (8), whereas in young men aged 18 to 24 years, the reported incidence of UTIs is 0.01 per person-year (9). The incidence of UTIs decreases in middle age but increases in older adults (10–12).

More than 10% of women over 65 years of age reported having had a urinary tract infection in the past 12 months (11). This figure rises to almost 30% among women over 85 years of age (12).

In a large prospective cohort study of community-dwelling postmenopausal women, the incidence of UTI was 0.07 per person-year and 0.12 per person-year in older women with diabetes (10).

For men aged 65 to 74 years, the incidence of urinary tract infections is estimated at 0.05 per person-year (9).

In men and women over 85 years of age, the incidence of UTIs increases dramatically. A small cohort study in this age group found that the incidence of UTIs in women was 0.13 per person-year and 0.08 per person-year in men (13).

In our study, the mean age was 75.6 ± 6.5 years (65 to 97 years) and the most affected age group was adults aged between 65 and 80 years. We noted a female predominance (52.6%).

1.2. Incidence of asymptomatic bacteriuria in the elderly

BAS is more common in older adults than in younger adults. The prevalence increases dramatically with age in both men and women. In younger women, the estimated prevalence of BAS is 1–5%, increasing to approximately 6–16% in women over 65 years of age (2,14,15). In community-dwelling women over 80 years of age, the incidence is estimated to be nearly 20% (16).

In long-term care facilities, the prevalence is even higher, with estimates among women ranging from 25% to 50% (3).

In young ambulatory men, BAS is rare with prevalence rates reported between 0 and 1.5% (17); however, in men over 80 years of age, the prevalence is estimated to increase to nearly 10% (16).

Among aging men residing in long-term care facilities, the prevalence of BAS approaches that of women, ranging from 15 to 35% (3).

Urinary catheter use predisposes both men and women to BAS . The risk in catheterized elderly individuals ranges from 3 to 10% per day of catheterization, ultimately reaching 100% in adults with chronic indwelling catheters (14,18).

2. RISK FACTORS ASSOCIATED WITH URINARY TRACT INFECTIONS IN THE ELDERLY

Risk factors for developing symptomatic UTI in the aging population are different from those in younger women. Age-associated changes in immune function, exposure to nosocomial pathogens, and an increasing number of comorbidities place older adults at increased risk of developing infection (19).

2.1. Elderly people living in the community

Several risk factors associated with UTIs in postmenopausal women have been identified, many of which are similar to those in younger sexually active women. The most consistent and strong predictor across all age groups is having a history of UTI (10,20,21). In one study, postmenopausal women with a prior UTI were four times more likely to develop a subsequent UTI than women without a prior diagnosis (20). Women with more than six lifetime UTIs had a more than seven-fold increased risk of developing a subsequent UTI compared with women without a history of UTI (10). Diagnosis of UTI, particularly before age 15, has also been shown to increase risk in postmenopausal women, suggesting that genetic factors may predispose some women to recurrent infections (21).

2.2. Sexual activity

The relationship between sexual activity and UTIs is well established in younger women, although the association in postmenopausal women is not as clear. During sexual intercourse, vaginal bacteria gain access to the urinary tract by colonizing the periurethral mucosa and ascending to the bladder through the urethra (22).

A 2008 cohort study by Moore et al. reported an increased risk of developing UTI in postmenopausal women who reported having intercourse 2 days before symptom onset (hazard ratio, 3.42; 95% CI, 1.49 to 7.80). This increased risk of UTI was not demonstrated in women reporting intercourse 1 day before (hazard ratio, 1.01; 95% CI, 0.30 to 3.37) or >2 days before (hazard ratio, 0.95; 95% CI, 0.52 to 1.72), making the clinical significance of this finding unclear (23). Although up to 65% of postmenopausal women report being sexually active (24), most studies have not consistently found sexual intercourse to be a significant predictor of UTI in this population (10,21,23).

2.3. Urinary tract obstruction

One of the factors promoting urinary tract infection is obstruction of the urinary tract, allowing bacteria to adhere to urothelial cells. Thus, colonization of the perineum, vagina and urethral mucosa by uropathogenic strains constitutes a reservoir of germs responsible for cystitis (17,18).

2.4. Urinary retention

Urinary retention and elevated post-void residual urine (PVR) have been postulated to be a risk factor for UTI in the elderly. In men, prostatic hypertrophy causing obstruction of normal urinary flow results in elevated PVR. Elevated PVR and urinary stasis resulting from chronic obstruction are thought to be important factors for the development of UTI and BAS in elderly men; however, studies evaluating the association in this population are limited. In women, the association between elevated PVR and UTI has been more extensively examined, although data from several studies have yielded conflicting results. A 2011 cohort study of postmenopausal women did not find that high PROM (>200 mL) increased the risk of UTI at 1 year in a multivariate analysis, although PROM >200 mL was associated with more frequent urinary symptoms (25).

2.5. Institutionalized elderly persons

Institutionalized adults have functional impairments, higher rates of cognitive deficits, and more medical comorbidities than community-dwelling older adults. All of these characteristics predispose this population to higher rates of BAS and UTI (26). The most important risk factors associated with UTI in institutionalized older adults are the presence of a urinary catheter and, as in community-dwelling older adults, a history of UTI (3,13,27). Medical comorbidities, such as stroke and dementia, which can predispose individuals to bowel and bladder incontinence, have been associated with symptomatic UTI and persistent BAS in this population (13,26). Other predictors include disability in activities of daily living and a history of urinary incontinence (13). As in community women, elevated PROM was not associated with UTIs in nursing home residents (28). BAS , which is more common in nursing home residents and catheterized adults, was associated with an increased risk of symptomatic UTIs in a few studies (10,29).

2.6. Personal background

Diabetes is a contributing factor to urinary tract infection. Diabetes exposes the patient to the occurrence of urinary tract infection through the bladder residue caused by peripheral neuropathy. The presence of sugar in the urine promotes bacterial proliferation and impairs polymorphonuclear function. Cachexia and protein -energy malnutrition reduce the lymphocyte response as well as the secretory IgA level (34).

In the literature, urinary tract infections are favored by age with bladder motility disorders, dehydration, poor hygiene and decreased immune defenses (35). But there was no significant relationship between the occurrence of urinary tract infection and age.

In our study, personal history was noted in 312 cases (81.7%) dominated by diabetes (50.5%), high blood pressure (45%) and stroke (9.4%). The most common nephro -urological history was acute pyelonephritis (23.8%) and urinary stones (14.7%).

3. DIAGNOSIS OF URINARY TRACT INFECTIONS IN THE ELDERLY

Urinary tract infections in healthy older women without urinary catheters or genitourinary tract abnormalities are considered at risk for complications (30).

Diagnosis does not follow the same algorithm used in younger patients, requiring the presence of genitourinary symptoms and a positive urine culture. Common urinary symptoms suggestive of cystitis include urgency, urinary frequency, dysuria, and suprapubic tenderness. However, postmenopausal women may also present with nonspecific generalized symptoms, such as lower abdominal pain, back pain, chills, and constipation (24).

As with other populations, the diagnosis of symptomatic UTI in nursing home residents requires the presence of genitourinary symptoms in the setting of a positive urine culture. In older adults with intact cognitive function, the diagnosis of symptomatic UTI is relatively straightforward. However, nursing home residents often have significant cognitive deficits, impairing their ability to communicate, and chronic genitourinary symptoms (e.g., incontinence, urgency, and urinary frequency), which make the diagnosis of symptomatic UTI in this group particularly difficult. In addition, when infected, nursing home residents are more likely to present with nonspecific symptoms, such as anorexia, confusion, and decline in functional status (33). Fever may be absent or diminished (19). In the context of atypical symptoms, practitioners are often challenged in differentiating symptomatic UTI from other infections or medical problems. The high prevalence of bacteriuria and pyuria in this population often leads to the diagnosis of UTI. Although bacteriuria and pyuria are necessary for the diagnosis of laboratory-confirmed UTI, they are not sufficient alone to diagnose symptomatic UTI. To date, there are no universally accepted criteria for diagnosing UTI in this population, making it difficult for clinicians to distinguish symptomatic UTI from other conditions in the presence of new nonspecific symptoms (34).

To assist clinicians in diagnosing symptomatic UTIs, several consensus guidelines have been published, standardizing definitions of symptomatic UTIs in long-term care facilities. In 2001, Loeb et al. proposed a set of guidelines to assist practitioners in clinical decision making by providing recommendations on the minimum criteria necessary for initiating antibiotic treatment in nursing home residents (34). Loeb's criteria for diagnosing UTIs are presented in Table XX.

In 2012, members of the Society for Healthcare Epidemiology of America (SHEA) met to update the current guidelines. Significant changes were made to the definition of UTI for residents with and without urinary catheters. Specifically, the new definitions require a positive urine culture in residents with and without indwelling urinary catheters, or a positive blood and urine culture in residents without localized symptoms of UTI (37).

Although the guidelines proposed by Loeb et al. are commonly accepted, application of these criteria to clinical practice in the nursing home population is challenging and antibiotic overuse remains a significant problem. A major challenge clinicians face when diagnosing UTIs is the relatively low frequency of localized genitourinary symptoms (i.e., dysuria, pollakuria , and urgency) observed in nursing home residents, many of which are necessary components of the Loeb criteria (36).

Table XX presents a comparison of 2 published consensus definitions. The diagnostic accuracy of these guidelines has not yet been validated.

Table V: Comparison of consensus criteria for the diagnosis of symptomatic urinary tract infection in residents with and without an indwelling urinary catheter .

	SHEA/CDC 2012 (37) (criteria McGeer revised)	Loeb criteria (34)

Without indwelling urinary catheter	Must include criteria 1 and 2:
	1. At least one of the following signs or symptoms:
	• Acute dysuria or pain, swelling or tenderness of the testicles, epididymis or prostate or :
	• Fever or leukocytosis and at least one of the following symptoms or :
	  - Acute pain or tenderness at the costovertebral angle
	  - Suprapubic pain
	  - Macroscopic hematuria
	  - New or marked increase in incontinence
		Acute dysuria alone or :
		Fever (>37.9° or increase of 1.5°C from baseline) plus one of the following:
		
		- New or worsening urgency
		- Pollakiuria
		- Suprapubic pain
		- Macroscopic hematuria
		- Costovertebral angle sensitivity
		- Urinary incontinence

	- New or marked increase in urgency or pollakiuria • In the absence of fever and leukocytosis, at least two of the following: - Suprapubic pain - Macroscopic hematuria - New or marked increase in incontinence - New or marked increase in urgency - New or marked increase in pollakiuria 2. At least one of the following microbiological criteria: • $\geq 10^5$ CFU/ml, no more than two bacteria in a urine sample • $\geq 10^2$ CFU/ml of any number of organisms in a sample collected by minute sampling	
With an indwelling urinary catheter	One of the following criteria: - Fever, chills or new hypotension - Acute change in mental status or acute functional decline and leukocytosis - New onset suprapubic pain or costovertebral angle pain or tenderness - Purulent discharge around the catheter or sharp pain, swelling or tenderness in the testicles, epididymis or prostate + Positive urine culture (At least 10^5 CFU/ml of any organism)	At least one of the following: - Fever (> 37.9° or increase of 1.5°C compared to the initial value) - New costovertebral sensitivity - Rigors (trembling shivers) - New appearance of delirium

SHEA: Society for Healthcare Epidemiology in America.

In a study of nursing home residents with advanced dementia, change in mental status was the most common reason for suspected UTI, accounting for more than 40% of cases; localized genitourinary symptoms were uncommon. Dysuria accounted for only 3.8% of suspected cases, urinary frequency for 1.5% of cases, and no suspected UTI was due to urgency or suprapubic pain (38).

Furthermore, nearly 85% of suspected UTIs did not meet the criteria for initiation of antimicrobial therapy; however, most cases (75%) were treated with antibiotics (38). This study shows that, although criteria exist to help clinicians diagnose and treat UTIs, health care workers caring for this population may be reluctant to follow them. Furthermore, it highlights the overall low prevalence of typical genitourinary symptoms in severely demented patients with suspected UTIs (38).

A cohort study of nursing home residents attempted to identify clinical features predictive of bacteriuria and pyuria. Although bacteriuria and pyuria alone do not diagnose symptomatic UTI, their presence signifies a host inflammatory response to a microbial pathogen, both of which are necessary components in the diagnosis of UTI. The most commonly reported clinical features of suspected UTI in this cohort were change in mental status (39%), change in behavior (19%), change in urine character i.e. gross hematuria, and change in urine color or odor. (15.5%), fever or chills (12.8%) and change in gait or fall (8.8%) (39).

Although caregivers commonly report change in mental status and change in behavior, only three measures of mental status (i.e., periods of altered perception, disorganized speech, and lethargy) and one measure of behavior (i.e., resistance to care) have been shown to be effective when reliably assessed by caregivers caring for nursing home residents (40).

In a multivariate analysis, change in mental status, dysuria, and change in urine character were significantly associated with the development of bacteriuria and pyuria. Dysuria alone predicted 39% of cases of confirmed bacteriuria and pyuria; however, in combination with change in mental status or change in urine character, the predicted probability increased to 63% (39). This predicted probability is higher than the Loeb criteria, which had a positive predictive value of 57% for the detection of bacteriuria plus pyuria (41).

When all three clinical features were present, the predicted probability increased to 100%, but all three clinical features were present in only four episodes of suspected UTI. This suggests that a combination of nonspecific and urinary tract-specific symptoms (e.g., change in mental status, change in urine character, and dysuria) may be useful in the clinical assessment of nursing home residents with UTI (39,41). However, nonspecific symptoms, when present alone, have not been shown to correlate with bacteriuria (42).

Falls are common in older adults and often result in empiric antibiotic use when UTI is suspected. Although falls have been associated with UTI in a few studies, a recent report found that 80% of fall episodes were not associated with bacteriuria plus pyuria (43,44).

The diagnosis of UTI remains a significant diagnostic dilemma for clinicians caring for older adults. Fever and localized urinary symptoms should always be the first trigger for evaluation of UTI. According to the Infectious Diseases guidelines Disease Society of America, the minimum laboratory evaluation for suspected UTI should include a urinalysis for leukocyte esterase and nitrite using a dipstick, and microscopy for white blood cells. If the urine dipstick is negative for leukocyte esterase and nitrite in a nursing home resident, the negative predictive value is 100% and the evaluation can be discontinued (45).

In case of pyuria or presence of leukocyte esterase or nitrites, a urine culture should be performed and, if positive, antibiotic therapy should be considered if a urinary tract infection is suspected (33).

McGeer criteria , SHEA incorporates the use of a urine dipstick for leukocyte esterase and nitrite testing as part of the initial evaluation of suspected UTIs, consistent with the recommendations of the Infectious Diseases Disease Society of America (33).

4. CLINICAL DATA

4.1. Functional signs

Specific signs and symptoms of UI are more common in the healthy, independent older population (37). These specific symptoms are:

- ❖ Temperature $\geq 38.5°C$ or hypothermia $\leq 36.5°C$
- ❖ Dysuria, pollakiuria,
- ❖ urination ,

❖ Hematuria,

❖ Suprapubic tension,

❖ New onset urinary incontinence.

The institutionalized patient may also present with specific signs and symptoms; however, these elderly subjects may have atypical presentations of infection (30,37-40). These nonspecific or atypical symptoms include:

❖ Drowsiness,

❖ Appearance or worsening of anorexia,

❖ Appearance or worsening of disorientation,

❖ Fall,

❖ Appearance or worsening of dependency,

❖ Decompensation of a comorbidity.

Additionally, the inability to communicate with caregivers for more debilitated patients (stroke or dementia patients) and the presence of multiple comorbidities add to the diagnostic challenge in this population (38).

Workup of patients with atypical findings should include assessment of genitourinary signs or symptoms. Because BAS is common in this age group, a positive urine culture is not diagnostic (40).

The urinary tract is the most common source of bacteremia in institutionalized patients, with more than 50% being associated with organic/functional urinary tract abnormalities or indwelling urinary catheters (41).

Patients with pyelonephritis may present with signs consistent with sepsis (8).

Patients should be questioned about underlying conditions that may suggest the presence of complicated pyelonephritis (42).

Physical examination should include vital signs and assessment of signs and symptoms of acute pyelonephritis (37).

4.2. Clinical forms

In our study, acute pyelonephritis was the most observed clinical form (84.8%). While in other studies, asymptomatic bacteriuria and cystitis were the most observed clinical forms (Table XXI).

Table XXI: Clinical forms in the literature

Clinical forms	Barrier (59)	Fongoro (61)	Haber (55)	Our study
Acute pyelonephritis	15%	25.6%	32.9%	84.8%
Cystitis	13%	24.3%	56.7%	6.3%
Prostatitis	15%	9.7%	9.4%	5%
Asymptomatic bacteriuria	21%	40.2%	-	-

This difference is explained by the fact that our population included mainly patients who were hospitalized.

Barrier (59) reported 41% asymptomatic bacteriuria. Several studies have shown that bacteriuria is more common in women than in men and its frequency increases with age in both sexes. Between 65 and 70 years 20% of women and 2-3% of men have bacteriuria and after 80 years 23-50% of women and 20% of men (47-51).

4.3. Signs of severity

Elderly subjects, especially bedridden ones, frequently have acute pyelonephritis, whether they have prostatic hypertrophy or have no urological abnormalities. The signs are often serious: 30% of septicemias in elderly subjects are of urinary origin, especially in hospital settings. The diagnosis may not be made quickly due to the absence of lower back pain or impaired consciousness. Any fever in a bedridden elderly person should, among other tests, motivate a urine culture . The development of these urinary septicemias in elderly patients is quite often fatal, especially if it is not thought of and if treatment is delayed (22).

In the study of López -Cruz (32), septic shock at presentation was found in 17.4% of patients and urosepsis in 57.8% of patients. There was no significant association between polymicrobial infection and septic shock in men (p = 0.123).

Furthermore, López -Cruz (32) noted that male gender was associated with septic shock (24.29% versus 12.09% in women, p = 0.043). This prevalence of more severe forms of infections in men was described in a large Korean study of patients with sepsis from different health facilities, where it was found that organ failure was more frequent in men, although septic shock was similar in both sexes (33). In addition, another Italian study showed that men present septic shock more often and are younger than women in intensive care (34).

Ioannou 's study (35), sepsis and septic shock were the clinical presentation in 47% and 3% respectively, which was similar to other studies (6,17,18).

These rates were similar to the data from our study. We noted that a Systemic inflammatory response syndrome (SIRS) was the most common sign of severity (47.4%) and septic shock was noted in 1.6% of patients.

In a study in patients with acute pyelonephritis, concomitant bacteremia was noted in 19.4% of patients (18).

This percentage is close to that found in our study. More precisely, a blood culture was positive in 16.5% of patients. *Escherichia Coli* was the most isolated germ (53.9%) followed by *Klebsiella Pneumoniae* (19%).

While in other studies, including both older and younger patients, where blood cultures were performed in all patients, concomitant bacteremia ranged from 31 to 50% (17-19); however, older patients appeared more likely to develop bacteremia (17).

5. BACTERIOLOGICAL DATA

The most common organism causing UTIs and bacteremia in the community and health care settings is *Escherichia coli*, followed by other Enterobacteriaceae, such as *Proteus mirabilis, Klebsiella, and Providencia* species. Gram-positive organisms, such as *Staphylococcus aureus* and methicillin-resistant *Enterococcus* , are less common overall but are increasingly being seen in health care settings and in adults with chronic indwelling catheters (46,47).

The germs involved are most often of endogenous origin and colonize the urinary tract by ascending rather than hematogenous route. *Escherichia Coli* is the most common germ (80%) and is of fecal origin (20, 29). *Staphylococcus saprophyticus* (10 to 30%) is a commensal germ of the skin and genital tract (20). Other gram-negative bacilli (GNB) such as *Klebsiella* , *Proteus* , *Enterobacter* and *Pseudomonas* are mainly found in patients with predisposing factors (immunodepression, hospital stay, catheterization, etc.) (30).

Haber and Coudert reported Gram-negative bacilli in 88.5% and 83.6% of cases, respectively (55,56). The predominance of *Escherichia coli* in urine culture was reported by Haber (55) and Coudert (56) with 51.6% and 59.7% of cases, respectively. Barrier reported 37% of *E. coli* (59).

In the study by López -Cruz (32), Escherichia *coli was* the most common cause of infection (60.9%). The rate of polymicrobial infection was 11.2% and was higher in men than in women (6.6% vs. 17.1%, respectively; p = 0.035). The rate of *Pseudomonas aeruginosa infection* was 9.3% and statistically higher in men (3.3% in women vs. 17.1% in men; p = 0.003).

In our study, of the 366 positive cultures (95.8%), *Escherichia coli* was the most isolated germ (57.6%). Contaminated urine was noted in only one patient (0.3%). Leukocyturia was present in 358 patients (93.7%).

The age-specific distribution of pathogenic bacteria in UTIs is another crucial area of investigation (12). Age has been associated with the incidence of UTIs and treatment failure of UTIs in many observational studies, sometimes with conflicting results (13–15). Therefore, knowing how the incidence of UTIs varies across different age groups can contribute to the development of targeted prevention strategies and tailored therapeutic approaches, taking into account the unique physiological and immunological characteristics of specific populations (16,17).

A better understanding of the factors contributing to the development and spread of UTIs can pave the way for the implementation of effective public health measures, including educational campaigns to raise awareness of preventive practices and hygiene habits (18). Community-wide efforts can thus foster a culture of proactive health management, ultimately reducing the incidence of UTIs and improving the overall quality of life of individuals worldwide (2,19).

The present study highlights the distribution of bacterial pathogens in UTIs with respect to seasonality, sex, and age. The predominant bacterial pathogens identified were *E. coli* (50.0%), *E. faecium* (15.6%), *E. faecalis* (9.6%), *K. pneumoniae* (6.8%), *P. aeruginosa* (3.5%), *A. baumannii* (2.7 %), *S. agalactiae* (2.5%), *S. aureus* (2.1%), and *P. mirabilis* (1.2%). These results are consistent with those of previous studies (24-26). Another similar study by Faine et al (27) showed that among patients with positive urine cultures, 84.7% had cultures containing Enterobacteriaceae, with *E. coli* (62.8%) being the most frequently isolated pathogen (27-30).

The study of seasonal distribution revealed a significant association between specific bacterial species and particular seasons. Notably, *E. faecium* showed higher prevalence in spring and *A. baumannii* in autumn (9).

These data are consistent with a previous study by Alrashid et al (31), which also demonstrated a seasonal trend, with the highest number of confirmed UTIs in January and the lowest in April.

This complexity adds to our understanding of UTIs and highlights the need to consider seasonal variations when developing diagnostic and preventive strategies, as supported by the previous study by Simmering et al (8).

Analysis of the sex distribution revealed notable differences in the prevalence of bacterial pathogens between male and female groups. Urinary tract infections were much more common in women than in men due to certain anatomical and physiological characteristics, such as a shorter urethra, proximity of the urethral orifice to the anus, changes during menopause, pregnancy and other factors, with this difference increasing with age (34,35).

Men with UTIs had a higher susceptibility to Gram-positive bacterial infections than their female counterparts (35.9% vs. 26.9%; p = 0.004). *E. faecalis* , *S. aureus* , *P. aeruginosa* , and *A. baumannii* showed a significant difference between sexes, being more common in men.

Silva et al (36) observed a higher prevalence of urinary tract infections caused by *E. faecalis* and *P. aeruginosa* in men than in women (8.8% for *E. faecalis* and 8.1% for *P. aeruginosa* in men, versus 1.8 and 1.6% in women).

A study by Magliano et al (37) demonstrated that *P. aeruginosa* and *E. faecalis* were more frequently found in men than in women (p < 0.05).

Amna et al (38) determined that non-E. coli bacteria were more likely to infect men, citing the increased complexity of UTIs in men, often attributed to frequent catheter use (39,40).

Specifically, *Enterococcus* and *Pseudomonas* have been associated with catheter-associated urinary tract infections (41,42). These findings highlight the complex interplay between biological, anatomical, and behavioral factors in the prevalence of UTIs.

The higher frequency of Gram-positive bacteria in men suggests the possibility of sex-related disparities in immunity or physiological factors that may make men more susceptible to UTIs (11,43). The results of these studies, showing an increase in *S. aureus* in men, are consistent with research by Stokes et al (44), who demonstrated a higher prevalence of *S. aureus* in men, particularly in older age groups with comorbidities. Understanding sex-specific variations in bacterial prevalence holds promise for targeted interventions and awareness campaigns tailored to each sex group (45).

By addressing the unique factors that influence UTIs in men and women, progress can be made toward reducing UTI rates and improving overall health outcomes (46).

The present study on the age distribution of bacterial pathogens revealed significant associations between some species and different age groups. The study highlighted that Gram-positive bacteria, particularly *E. faecium*, showed a marked increase in prevalence in older people with urinary tract infections. These results are consistent with those of previous studies (47,48).

The notable age-related associations observed for *E. coli* in the present study showed a higher prevalence in younger individuals with UTIs. These age-related patterns of bacterial pathogens add a new layer of complexity to our understanding of UTIs. The substantial changes in bacterial prevalence of UTIs with age underscore the importance of age-specific management strategies that lead to better health care outcomes (49,50).

6. TREATMENT

Urinary tract infections are the most common indication for antibiotic prescription in older adults. Choosing the right antibiotic and the duration of antibiotic treatment are two important issues to consider when treating UTIs in older adults. Previous studies have demonstrated that 40% to 75% of antimicrobial use is inappropriate (38,48).

Overuse of antibiotics leads to negative consequences, including the development of multidrug-resistant organisms, adverse side effects (such as Clostridium difficile infection), and high healthcare costs. Differentiating symptomatic UTIs from BAS remains particularly challenging, and treatment of BAS remains a common reason for antimicrobial prescription (46).

6.1. Antibiotic therapy

The choice of antibiotic should fundamentally be personalized and adapted to each elderly patient. The selection should be taken into account based on bacterial pathogens, antibiotic resistance rates, side effects, and comorbidities of the patients. Generally, an antibiotic with high urinary excretion levels is recommended in the treatment of UTIs (30).

Once a UTI with fever is diagnosed, empirical antimicrobial therapy should be initiated to prevent progression to sepsis or even septic shock. The decision to indicate a broad-spectrum antibiotic should be based on the severity of the infection, the presence of known risk factors, and local rates of antimicrobial resistance. Increasing carbapenem consumption has been identified as a factor in the acquisition of carbapenemase among Enterobacteriaceae strains (36).

Given the high frequency of antimicrobial resistance in elderly patients with UTIs, it would be advisable to consider local microbiology and resistance patterns when choosing antimicrobials for these infections, as has also been suggested in the literature. The development of local protocols for antimicrobial selection based on local antimicrobial resistance patterns may lead to more effective and accurate treatment of these infections (29).

6.1.1. Cystitis
6.1.1.1. Cystitis at risk of complication

A cytobacteriological examination must be carried out after a urine orientation strip (37).

According to the Tunisian recommendations for antibiotic therapy for urinary tract infections: If treatment cannot be postponed, while waiting for the antibiogram, probabilistic treatment is based on Nitrofurantoin (100 mg x 3/day) or Pivmecillinam (400 mg x 2/day) or fosfomycin- trometamol (3 g/day 1 day/2 x 3 doses).

If treatment can be delayed by 24-48 hours, the initial antibiotic therapy would be adapted to the antibiogram

❖ 1st choice: amoxicillin 1 gx 3/day (DTT = 7 days)

❖ 2nd choice: Pivmecillinam 400 mg x 2/day (DTT = 7 days)

Or Nitrofurantoin 100 mg x 3/day (DTT = 7 days)

Or TMP-SMX (80mg/400mg) 2 tabs x 2 / day

❖ 3rd choice: fosfomycin- tromethamine 3 doses of 3 g on D1 - D3 - D5

Or Amoxicillin -clavulanic acid 1g*3/day

6.1.2. Pyelonephritis

6.1.2.1. Pyelonephritis at risk of complication

Referring to Tunisian recommendations, probabilistic antibiotic therapy for PNA without signs of severity is based on parenteral C3G (Cefotaxime 1g x 3/day IV or IM and ceftriaxone 1g/day IV or IM).

For oral relay treatment after bacteriological documentation and in order of least effect on the microbiota, we can use:

❖ Amoxicillin 1g x 3/day

❖ Cotrimoxazole 2cp x 2 /day

❖ Amoxicillin -clavulanic acid 1g x 3/day

❖ Fluoroquinolone (ciprofloxacin 500mg x 2/day)

❖ Cefixime 200 mg x 2/day

The processing time would be 10 to 14 days for C3G.

The duration of treatment is only 7 days if parenteral C3G or fluoroquinolones have been used as a relay.

6.1.2.2. Severe pyelonephritis

Treatment is based on a combination of C3G (Cefotaxime or ceftriaxone) with an aminoside (amikacin) with a high dosage in the absence of risk factors for nephrotoxicity. In case of allergy to Beta-lactam: Amikacin + Fosfomycin or Amikacin + Colimycin are combined .

Note that the FDRs of aminoglycoside nephrotoxicity are presented by:

❖ Advanced age > 75 years

❖ Concomitant use of other nephrotoxic drugs or iodinated contrast agents

❖ Dehydration

❖ Renal failure (Creatinine clearance < 60 ml/min)

❖ Pre-existing or concomitant nephropathy

❖ Severe cirrhosis grade B and C according to the Child- Pugh classification

❖ Taking medications that promote renal hypoperfusion (loop diuretics, angiotensin converting enzyme inhibitors or angiotensin II antagonists, nonsteroidal anti-inflammatory drugs).

The processing time is 10 to 14 days.

6.1.2.3. Severe pyelonephritis with FDR of BLSE

The BLSE FDRs are presented by:

❖ Recent use of antibiotics,

❖ Hospitalization within 3 months or being in a long-stay facility

❖ The presence of an indwelling catheter

❖ And the recent trip to an area where BLSE is endemic

❖ A history of digestive or urinary colonization with EBLSE has been considered by some authors as a risk factor.

In these cases, the recommended dual therapy would be Imipenem + Amikacin.

For oral relay

❖ 1st choice

> Fluoroquinolones S: ofloxacin, ciprofloxacin

> Fluoroquinolones R and cotrimoxazole S: Cotrimoxazole

> Fluoroquinolones R and cotrimoxazole R and amoxicillin-clavulanic acid S: Amoxicillin-clavulanic acid

> Fluoroquinolones R, Cotrimoxazole -R and amikacin S: Amikacin

❖ 2nd choice

> Piperacillin -Tazobactam S: Piperacillin tazobactam

❖ 3rd choice

> Ertapenem

6.1.3. Male IU

6.1.3.1. Male UI without signs of severity

Paucisymptomatic male urinary tract infection may not require probabilistic antibiotic therapy and treatment may be deferred based on microbiological documentation. According to the recommendations, poorly tolerated male UTI or the presence of associated fever indicates the prescription of Cefotaxime or ceftriaxone.

Note that FQs and cotrimoxazole are the two molecules of choice for the relay.

The minimum recommended duration is:

❖ In pauci-symptomatic forms without associated uropathy: 14 days.

❖ In the presence of underlying uropathy, an associated risk factor for complications or in the case of use of an antibiotic other than fluoroquinolone or cotrimoxazole: 21 days.

6.1.3.2. Male UI with sign of severity

This infection is considered identical to severe PNA and therefore the treatment would be the same as that indicated for severe PNA.

6.1. 3.3. Recurrent cystitis

The treatment of recurrent cystitis in the elderly is essentially based on hygiene and dietary rules, mainly good hydration, not retaining urine, not using excessive toilet products and wearing cotton underwear.

Antibiotic prophylaxis should only be recommended when cystitis recurs despite strict application of the measures detailed above. It allows a reduction in the frequency of cystitis.

The antibiotics used are cotrimoxazole (trimethoprim - sulfamethoxazole) or fosfomycin - trometamol .

It should be remembered that the objective of antibiotic prophylaxis is not the sterilization of urine. Control by ECBU under antibiotic prophylaxis is then not indicated.

Possible protocols:

❖ Recurrent cystitis ≥ 1 time/month: SMX + TMP (400/80): 1 tablet /day or 1 tablet/day 3 days/week to be taken in the evening at bedtime Or Fosfomycin- tromethamine : 3g/7 – 10 days

❖ Post-coital cystitis: the same antibiotics must be taken within 2 hours before or after intercourse without exceeding the curative doses: SMX+TMP (400/80): 1 tablet Or Fosfomycin- tromethamine : 3g (maximum 1 x / 7 days).

6.1.4. Urinary tract infections on indwelling catheters

Many frail elderly patients require long-term urethral catheterization, with approximately 5–10% of residents in long-term care facilities relying on chronic indwelling catheters for bladder drainage. Special consideration should be given to the management of urinary tract infections in this patient group. In patients with an indwelling catheter in situ for more than 1 week, the urethral catheter should ideally be changed before the urine sample is collected for culture. This has been shown to reduce the incidence of catheter biofilm contamination. It has also been shown to allow rapid defervescence and reduced symptomatic relapses after treatment in patients with long-term urethral catheters (50).

It is strongly recommended to initiate probabilistic antibiotic therapy within one hour of diagnosis of severe sepsis.

It is strongly recommended to start probabilistic antibiotic therapy within 12 hours following the diagnosis of parenchymal infection (pyelonephritis, prostatitis, epididymo- orchitis).

In other situations, in the absence of comorbidity favoring serious infections or risk situations, it is strongly recommended to postpone antibiotic therapy in order to adapt it to the results of the urine culture (51).

However, the optimal duration of antimicrobial therapy has not been evaluated, although it generally ranges from 5 to 21 days depending on the bacterial species, patient comorbidities, and patient response after initiation of treatment. Long-term suppressive antibiotic therapy in patients with long-term urethral catheters is not recommended because catheterized urine cannot be permanently sterilized (50).

6.2. Shortened antibiotic therapy in urinary tract infections

6.2.1. Cystitis at risk of complication

There is no new information in the literature regarding the duration of treatment of cystitis at risk of complications. The recommended antibiotic treatment is as follows (51):

- ❖ Trimethoprim/ sulfamethoxazole : 5 days
- ❖ Other molecules (except fluoroquinolones which are contraindicated in this case): 7 days

6.2.2 . Acute pyelonephritis

A 2020 meta-analysis by the Italian Society of Internal Medicine (52) on the optimal duration of antibiotic treatment for uncomplicated ANP concluded that short courses (7 days or less) were as effective as longer courses (7–14 days) when using FQs or C3Gs. For trimethoprim/ sulfamethoxazole (TMP/SMX), a 14-day course remains recommended.

A multicentre observational study conducted in England between 2010 and 2016 (53), including 272 women with *E. coli PNA* , showed that a 7-day course of ciprofloxacin was as effective as a 7-day course of TMP/SMX, suggesting that the usual duration of TMP/SMX treatment should be reduced from 14 to 7 days.

A prospective, multicenter, open-label, randomized French study (54), including 100 cases of uncomplicated PNA, compared a 5-day treatment with fluoroquinolones (Ofloxacin or Levofloxacin) to a 10-day treatment, and concluded that it was equivalent in terms of cure and risk of recurrence.

6.2.3. Male urinary tract infection

The concept of "cystitis in men" seems to be emerging and distinguishing itself from prostatitis tables. A retrospective English study (55) reports that 20% of elderly men with urinary tract infection (UTI) are prescribed antibiotic treatment of less than 7 days, suggesting that some clinicians are already opting for short treatments in a targeted male population.

A retrospective cohort analysis, based on a multicenter database of 573 male UTI records treated as outpatients (56), evaluated the impact of antibiotic choices and duration on the risk of recurrence. This study suggests that after excluding patients with complicating factors (parenchymal infection, signs of prostatitis, PNA, urinary tract abnormalities, uropathy, benign prostatic hyperplasia, lithiasis or immunosuppression), a treatment duration of 7 days is sufficient and is not associated with a higher risk of recurrence than longer treatments.

A large English analysis of a retrospective cohort of UTIs in men over 65 years of age (n = 33,745) compared outcomes across different durations of antibiotic treatment, ranging from 3 to 14 days (57). The findings indicate less toxicity of short courses with an increased risk of recurrence considered "acceptable" (1 recurrence per 150 infections).

Finally, a retrospective study of a cohort of 21,864 patients conducted in Denmark (58) concluded that a 5-day course of pivmecillinam (400 mg 3 times daily) is as effective as a 7-day course in preventing the risk of recurrence in the treatment of community-acquired low-grade UTI (" cystitis -like") due to *E. coli* in men over 70 years of age.

7. UNFAVORABLE DEVELOPMENT

In the study of Ioannou (35), 26.2% of survivors were readmitted to the hospital within 3 months. López -Cruz (32) reported 3 cases of relapse at 10 days.

In our patients, an unfavorable evolution was found in 81 patients (21.2%) and mortality was 3.1%.

In patients over 65 years of age, Ackermann (63) reported a mortality rate of 17% and Ioannou (35) a mortality of 17.6%.

In another study, Meyers (64) reported a 30% mortality rate in elderly patients when the source of bacteremia was the genitourinary tract.

The relatively higher mortality rate in these studies may be partly explained by the older age of their patients and the higher percentage of underlying disorders that have been shown to be an important risk factor in other studies (35, 63, 65).

Some studies have shown that advanced age is associated with increased mortality. The frequency and severity of underlying diseases increase with age. When comparing the influence of age and underlying diseases in bacteremic patients on mortality, age was not found to be an independent factor of poor prognosis. The interaction between advanced age and underlying diseases could impair functional status, reflecting reduced physiological reserve. This may be an important risk factor for mortality in critically ill elderly patients (63-67).

8. PREVENTION OF URINARY TRACT INFECTIONS

Prevention of UTIs in older adults is an important issue, as antibiotic overuse in this population remains high. Although many studies have focused on preventing symptomatic UTIs, prevention of BAS may also lead to decreased antibiotic use, particularly in nursing homes.

8.1. Elderly people in community and institutionalized settings

Strategies for preventing recurrent UTIs in postmenopausal women have been studied and include the use of antibiotic prophylaxis and nonantimicrobial therapies, such as estrogen replacement therapy and cranberry formulations. Estrogens are thought to play an important role in maintaining a low vaginal pH in premenopausal women. As estrogen levels decline in postmenopausal women, the vaginal flora changes and lactobacilli, the predominant flora in younger women, are often absent. This results in an increase in vaginal pH and promotes colonization of the vagina by uropathogens , such as *E. coli* (50). Intravaginal estrogen replacement has been shown in a few small studies to reduce the recurrence of UTIs in postmenopausal women (51,52), although oral estrogens do not (20,53). A recent Cochrane review concluded that vaginal estrogens have potential benefits in postmenopausal women with recurrent UTIs and symptoms of vaginal atrophy, although the evidence to support this recommendation is limited (54).

An oral formulation of lactobacilli was tested as a preventive strategy in postmenopausal women with recurrent UTI. The hypothesis was that oral lactobacilli could repopulate the vagina with premenopausal vaginal flora, thereby preventing UTIs. However, a randomized controlled trial evaluating the efficacy of oral lactobacilli found that oral lactobacilli were inferior to antibiotics in preventing recurrent UTIs. Furthermore, they found no evidence of lactobacilli in vaginal swabs, suggesting that treatment did not restore lactobacilli to the vaginal flora. However, they found a high rate of antibiotic-resistant isolates (>95%) after 1 month in women taking oral antibiotics (55). Intravaginal lactobacilli in premenopausal women have been shown to increase vaginal lactobacilli colonization and reduce the rate of recurrent UTIs by nearly 50% (relative risk, 0.5; 95% CI, 0.2–1.2), but these results were not statistically significant. The effect of intravaginal lactobacilli in postmenopausal women is unknown and warrants further study (56).

Cranberry formulations are another non-antimicrobial treatment used for the prevention of UTIs in the elderly. Cranberry proanthocyanidin (PAC) is the active ingredient in cranberry that inhibits the adhesion *of E. coli* fimbriated P to uroepithelial cells (57). A study by Avorn et al. demonstrated that among women living in nursing homes and assisted living facilities, 10 ounces (300 mL) of cranberry juice cocktail reduced bacteriuria and pyuria after 6 months of follow-up (58). A major limitation of this study was that participants in the placebo arm of the trial had a higher rate of prior UTIs (59). This study concluded that 10 ounces of cranberry juice cocktail, which contains 36 mg of PAC, may be effective in reducing bacteriuria and pyuria. However, subsequent studies in older adults using cranberry products (e.g., juice, capsules, or tablets) have yielded conflicting results. Therefore, there is little evidence to suggest the use of cranberry products in the prevention of symptomatic UTIs (60). Two major limitations of published studies of cranberry products are that older adults were unable to ingest the necessary amount of cranberry juice cocktail; or the capsules/tablets did not contain the 36 mg of PAC needed to demonstrate a potential benefit. Future studies should test cranberry products containing at least 36 mg of PAC to determine if they are effective in preventing bacteriuria, pyuria, and UTIs in older adults.

8.2. Catheterized patients

Catheter-associated bacteriuria is the most common infection in hospitals and long-term care facilities (31,61). The development of prevention strategies, including aseptic insertion of urinary catheters, minimization of catheter use, and minimization of catheter duration, has led to a decrease in the incidence of catheter-associated urinary tract infections (18).

In adults requiring catheterization, the use of antimicrobial-coated catheters may delay bacterial colonization and thereby decrease the incidence of catheter-associated UTIs. A recently published randomized controlled trial evaluated the use of two antibiotic-coated catheters (silver alloy-coated catheter and nitrofural -impregnated catheter) to reduce the incidence of symptomatic catheter-associated UTIs in patients requiring short-term catheter use. No benefit was seen with either catheter in preventing symptomatic UTIs. However, use of the nitrofural -impregnated catheter reduced the incidence of bacteriuria. This finding may have important implications, as the overuse of antibiotics to treat BAS remains a significant problem (62).

Proper catheter care to prevent unnecessary catheter-associated mechanical genitourinary injury and early identification of catheter obstruction help reduce the risk of UTI and potential subsequent systemic infections (68).

Antimicrobial-coated catheters have been reported to slightly decrease the risk of catheter-associated urinary tract infection, but are associated with more frequent catheter removal, catheter discomfort, and higher cost (69).

Chronic indwelling catheters do not need to be changed very frequently. Additional exchanges in addition to routine replacements are only necessary in cases of obstruction or symptomatic urinary tract infection after initiation of antimicrobial therapy (70).

Systemic antibiotic prophylaxis in patients with long-term urinary catheters does not reduce rates of bacteriuria, catheter-associated urinary tract infection, or death and should not be recommended (71).

When encountering patients with chronic indwelling catheters, clinicians should always question why a long-term urinary catheter was inserted in the first place and reassess regularly to reconsider whether it is still necessary and whether a trial without a catheter can be safely performed (72).

This reassessment may be useful especially for hospitalized patients to avoid urinary catheters beyond the expected necessary duration (73).

9. LIMITATIONS AND STRENGTHS OF THE PRESENT STUDY

⟂ Highlights:

❖ Clinical relevance:

Urinary tract infection in the elderly is a major public health problem due to the frequency of this pathology and the increased vulnerability of this population. Studying its clinical and therapeutic particularities will have a significant impact on management and improvement of care.

❖ Population specificity:

By focusing on elderly subjects, the thesis addresses a population often understudied in medical research, thereby filling important gaps in current knowledge in the absence of recommendations for this age group.

❖ **Contribution to medical practice:**

The findings of the thesis provide practical recommendations for clinicians, improve treatment protocols and potentially reduce morbidity and mortality rates related to urinary tract infections in the elderly.

❖ **Multidisciplinary approach:**

This thesis demonstrates the integration of geriatrics, microbiology, pharmacology and nursing aspects, thus providing a holistic perspective on the management of urinary tract infections in the elderly.

❖ **Sample size:**

The thesis uses a large sample size, which strengthens the reliability and validity of the results. A large sample allows for better generalization of the conclusions to the entire elderly population and increases the statistical robustness of the analyses.

✛ **Boundaries**

❖ **Variability of cases:**

Older adults often have varying comorbidities and health conditions, which may make it difficult to generalize the results of the thesis to the entire older population.

❖ Complexity of Treatments:

Treatment of urinary tract infections in older adults can be complicated by factors such as polypharmacy and antibiotic resistance, making therapeutic recommendations more complex to formulate.

❖ **Selection bias:**

There may be selection bias because the subjects studied come from hospital settings and have attended care settings, which may not reflect the situation of older people living independently.

10. RECOMMENDATIONS

⫩ Clinical Recommendations:

❖ **1. Early diagnosis and monitoring:**

Establish early diagnostic protocols to rapidly detect urinary tract infections in older people, particularly those who have attended care settings or have comorbidities.

❖ **2. Personalized support:**

Adapt treatments according to the clinical particularities of elderly patients, taking into account comorbidities, polymedication and possible resistance to antibiotics.

❖ **3. Rational use of antibiotics:**

Promote the rational use of antibiotics to avoid the development of resistance. Recommend treatments based on urine cultures and antibiograms for targeted prescription.

❖ **4. Hydration and hygiene:**

Encourage good hydration and adequate hygiene measures to prevent urinary tract infections. Educate patients and caregivers on the importance of these preventive measures.

⫩ Therapeutic Recommendations:

❖ **1. Choice of antibiotics:**

Select antibiotics that are appropriate for common resistance profiles in older adults. Prefer treatments with a good safety profile and low risk of drug interactions.

❖ **2. Monitoring and reassessment:**

Perform regular monitoring and reassessment of patients under treatment to adjust prescriptions based on clinical progress and laboratory test results.

❖ **3. Prophylaxis:**

Consider prophylactic measures for patients with recurrent UTIs, such as low-dose prophylactic antibiotics or use of non-antibiotic methods.

Institutional Recommendations:

❖ **1. Training of healthcare personnel:**

Train healthcare personnel in the recognition of atypical signs and symptoms of urinary tract infections in the elderly and in the appropriate management of these infections.

❖ **2. Standardized protocols:**

Develop and implement standardized management protocols for urinary tract infections in the elderly, based on the latest scientific evidence and best practice recommendations.

❖ **3. Continuous research:**

Encourage continued research on urinary tract infections in the elderly to improve knowledge and refine clinical and therapeutic recommendations.

By implementing these recommendations, we can hope for better management of urinary tract infections in the elderly, thereby reducing the associated morbidity and improving the quality of life of this population.

CONCLUSION

Urinary tract infections are the second most common cause of infection in the elderly, after respiratory tract infections.

Urinary tract infections are the leading causes of bacteremia, need for systemic antimicrobial therapy, hospitalization, decreased functional status, sepsis, and even death in frail elderly patients.

As part of the study of this pathology in elderly patients and to better support these particularities, we conducted a study with the following objectives:

- ❖ To study the epidemiological, clinical and paraclinical characteristics of urinary tract infection in the elderly.
- ❖ Detail the therapeutic management of this clinical entity.

To this end, we conducted a descriptive retrospective study of elderly patients hospitalized for a urinary tract infection in the infectious diseases department of the Hédi Chaker University Hospital in Sfax between January 2010 and December 2022.

During the 13 years of the study, we collected 382 cases of patients aged over 65 years who were followed for urinary tract infection with an average annual frequency of 29.4 cases/year (from 19 to 45 cases/year).

The mean age of our patients was 75.6 ± 6.5 years (range 65–97 years) and the most affected age group was adults aged 65–80 years.

We noted a female predominance (52.6%) with a male/female sex ratio equal to 0.9.

The 382 confirmed urinary tract infections were classified as community-acquired in 351 cases (91.9%) and nosocomial in the remaining 31 cases (8.1%).

For nosocomial infections, the infection appeared mainly during a stay in a hospitalization department (64.5%).

Acute pyelonephritis was the most observed clinical form (84.8%).

Systemic inflammatory response syndrome (SIRS) was the most common sign of severity (47.4%).

Among our patients, 81.2% were hospitalized with an average duration of 8 days (from 1 day to 2 months).

Escherichia *coli* was the most isolated germ (62.8%) .

The most common germs found in cases of nosocomial UTI were *Klebsiella pneumoniae* (n=12; 38.7%).

For the Enterobacteriaceae strains tested, we found a sensitivity to imipenem of 94.6% and to amikacin of 92%.

Compared to community infections, nosocomial infections were significantly due to multiresistant germs (77.4%).

Empirical antibiotic therapy was initiated in 68.8% of patients and documented antibiotic therapy in 30.1% of patients.

Empirical antibiotic therapy was then adapted according to the results of the antibiogram and the mean duration of antibiotic therapy was 16 ± 9 days with extremes from 1 to 36 days.

Radioguided drainage was performed in 1.8% of patients and surgical management was performed in 4.2% of patients.

A favorable evolution was noted in 75.6% of patients with a mean time to apyrexia of 2.1 ± 1.9 days (from 1 to 20 days).

An unfavorable evolution was found in 21.2% of patients and mortality was 3.1%.

Urinary tract infections and BAS are very common in older adults. Overuse of antibiotics for BAS remains a significant problem, particularly in long-term care facilities.

A major challenge facing clinicians is distinguishing symptomatic UTIs from BAS.

BIBLIOGRAPHY

1. Zeng G, Zhu W, Lam W, Bayramgil A. Treatment of urinary tract infections in the old and frail. World J Urol . 2020; 38(11):2709-20.

2. World Health Organization. Ageing and health. WHO, Geneva; 2022.

3. Teytaud M, Faraggi L. Urinary tract infections in the elderly: from diagnosis to the proper use of antibiotics. Le Pharmacien Hospitalier et Clinicien. 2017; 52(1):e21.

4. Caron F, Galperine T, Flateau C, Azria R, Bonacorsi S, Bruyère F, et al. Practice guidelines for the management of adult community-acquired urinary tract infections. Med Mal Infect. 2018; 48(5):327–58.

5. Pavese P.   Nosocomial urinary tract infections : definition, diagnosis, pathophysiology, prevention, treatment. Méd Mal Infect 2003; 33: 266-74.

6. Fried LP, Tangen CM, Walston J, Newman AB, Hirsch C, Gottdiener J, et al. Frailty in older adults: evidence for a phenotype. J Gerontol A Biol Sci Med Sci. 2001;56(3):146-56.

7. Singer M, Deutschman CS, Seymour CW, Shankar-Hari M, Annane D, Bauer M, et al. The Third International Consensus Definitions for Sepsis and Septic Shock (Sepsis-3). JAMA. 2016;315(8):801-10.

8. Kellum JA, Lameire N, Aspelin P, Barsoum RS, Burdmann EA, Goldstein SL, et al. Kidney disease: improving global outcomes (KDIGO) acute kidney injury work group. KDIGO clinical practice guideline for acute kidney injury. Kidney international supplements. 2012;2(1):1-138.

9. Stevens PE, Ahmed SB, Carrero JJ, Foster B, Francis A, Hall RK, et al. KDIGO 2024 Clinical Practice Guideline for the Evaluation and Management of Chronic Kidney Disease. Kidney International. 2024;105(4):117-314.

10. Jackson SL, Boyko EJ, Scholes D, Abraham L, Gupta K, Fihn SD. Predictors of urinary tract infection after menopause: a prospective study. Am J Med. 2004;117(12):903–911.

11. Foxman B, Barlow R, D'arcy H, Gillespie B, Sobel JD. Urinary tract infection: self-reported incidence and associated costs. Ann Epidemiol. 2000;10(8):509–515.

12. Eriksson I, Gustafson Y, Fagerstrom L, Olofsson B. Prevalence and factors associated with urinary tract infections (UTIs) in very old women. Arch Gerontol Geriatr . 2010;50(2):132–135.

13. Caljouw MA, Den Elzen WP, Cools HJ, Gussekloo J. Predictive factors of urinary tract infections among the oldest old in the general population. A population-based prospective follow-up study. BMC Med. 2011;9:57 .

14. Juthani -Mehta M. Asymptomatic bacteriuria and urinary tract infection in older adults. Clin Geriatr Med. 2007;23(3):585–594. vii.

15. Nicolle LE. Asymptomatic bacteriuria in the elderly. Infect Dis Clin North Am. 1997;11(3):647–662.

16. Rodhe N, Molstad S, Englund L, Svardsudd K. Asymptomatic bacteriuria in a population of elderly residents living in a community setting: prevalence, characteristics and associated factors. Family Pract . 2006;23(3):303–307.

17. Nicolle LE. Asymptomatic bacteriuria: when to screen and when to treat. Infect Dis Clin North Am. 2003;17(2):367–394.

18. Gould CV, Umscheid CA, Agarwal RK, Kuntz G, Pegues DA. Healthcare Infection Control Practices Advisory C Guideline for prevention of catheter-associated urinary tract infections 2009. Infect Control Hosp Epidemiol. 2010;31(4):319–326.

19. Juthani -Mehta M, Quagliarello VJ. Infectious diseases in the nursing home setting: challenges and opportunities for clinical investigation. Clin Infect Dis. 2010; 51(8):931–936.

20. Hu KK, Boyko EJ, Scholes D, et al. Risk factors for urinary tract infections in postmenopausal women. Arch Intern Med. 2004;164(9):989–993.

21. Raz R, Gennesin Y, Wasser J, et al. Recurrent urinary tract infections in postmenopausal women. Clin Infect Dis. 2000;30(1):152–156.

22. HootonTM. Clinical practice Uncomplicated urinary tract infection. N Engl J Med. 2012;366(11):1028–1037.

23. Moore EE, Hawes SE, Scholes D, Boyko EJ, Hughes JP, Fihn SD. Sexual intercourse and risk of symptomatic urinary tract infection in post-menopausal women. J Gen Intern Med. 2008;23(5):595–599.

24. Arinzon Z, Shabat S, Peisakh A, Berner Y. Clinical presentation of urinary tract infection (UTI) differs with aging in women. Arch Gerontol Geriatr . 2012;55(1):145–147.

25. Huang AJ, Brown JS, Boyko EJ, et al. Clinical significance of postvoid residual volume in older ambulatory women. J Am Geriatr Soc . 2011;59(8):1452–1458.

26. Eberle CM, Winsemius D, Garibaldi RA. Risk factors and consequences of bacteriuria in non-catheterized nursing home residents. J Gerontol . 1993;48(6):M266–M271.

27. Smith PW, Bennett G, Bradley S, et al. SHEA/APIC Guideline Infection prevention and control in the long-term care facility. Am J Infect Control. 2008;36(7):504–535.

28. Omli R, Skotnes LH, Mykletun A, Bakke AM, Kuhry E. Residual urine as a risk factor for lower urinary tract infection: a 1-year follow-up study in nursing homes. J Am Geriatr Soc. 2008;56(5):871–874.

29. Rodhe N, Lofgren S, Matussek A, et al. Asymptomatic bacteriuria in the elderly: high prevalence and high turnover of strains. Scand J Infect Dis. 2008;40(10):804–810.

30. Gupta K, Hooton TM, Naber KG, et al. International clinical practice guidelines for the treatment of acute uncomplicated cystitis and pyelonephritis in women: a 2010 update by the Infectious Diseases Society of America and the European Society for Microbiology and Infectious Diseases. Clin Infect Dis. 2011;52(5):e 103–e120.

31. Hooton TM, Bradley SF, Cardenas DD, et al. Diagnosis, prevention, and treatment of catheter-associated urinary tract infection in adults: 2009 International Clinical Practice Guidelines from the Infectious Diseases Society of America. Clin Infect Dis. 2010;50(5):625–663.

32. López-Cruz I, Esparcia A, Madrazo M, Alberola J, Eiros JM, Artero A. Sex differences in aged 80 and over hospitalized patients with community-acquired UTI: A prospective observational study. Heliyon . 2022;8(10):e 11131..

33. Park DW, Chun BC, Kim JM, Sohn JW, Peck KR, Kim YS, et al. Epidemiological and clinical characteristics of community-acquired severe sepsis and septic shock: a prospective observational study in 12 university hospitals in Korea. J Korean Med Sci. 2012;27(11):1308-14.

34. Sakr Y, Elia C, Mascia L, Barberis B, Cardellino S, Livigni S, et al. The influence of gender on the epidemiology of and outcome from severe sepsis. Crit Care. 2013;17(2):R 50.

35. Ioannou P, Plexousaki M, Dimogerontas K, Aftzi V, Drougkaki M, Konidaki M, et al. Characteristics of urinary tract infections in older patients in a tertiary hospital in Greece. Geriat Geront Int. 2020;20(12):1228-33.

36. Silva A, Costa E, Freitas A, Almeida A. Revisiting the frequency and antimicrobial resistance patterns of bacteria implicated in community urinary tract infections. Antibiotics (Basel) 2022; 11(768): 10-23.

37. Magliano E, Grazioli V, Deflorio L, Leuci AI, Mattina R, Romano P, Cocuzza CE. Gender and age-dependent etiology of community-acquired urinary tract infections. ScientificWorldJournal . 2012;2012(349597): 16-19.

38. Amna MA, Chazan B, Raz R, Edelstein H, Colodner R. Risk factors for non-Escherichia coli community-acquired bacteriuria. Infection. 2013;41:473-477 .

39. Prieto J, Wilson J, Bak A, Denton A, Flores A, Lusardi G, Reid M, Shepherd L, Whittome N, Loveday H. A prevalence survey of patients with indwelling urinary catheters on district nursing caseloads in the United Kingdom: The community urinary catheter management (CCaMa) study. J Infect Prev. 2020;21:129–135 .

40. Shackley DC, Whytock C, Parry G, Clarke L, Vincent C, Harrison A, John A, Provost L, Power M. Variation in the prevalence of urinary catheters: A profile of national health service patients in England. BMJ Open. 2017; 7:e013842 .

41. Gaston JR, Andersen MJ, Johnson AO, Bair KL, Sullivan CM, Guterman LB, White AN, Brauer AL, Learman BS, Flores-Mireles AL, Armbruster CE. Enterococcus faecalis polymicrobial interactions facilitate biofilm formation, antibiotic recalcitrance, and persistent colonization of the catheterized urinary tract. Pathogens. 2020;9(835): 10-23.

42. Lara-Isla A, Medina-Polo J, Alonso-Isa M, Benítez-Sala R, Sopeña-Sutil R, Justo- Quintas J, Gil - Moradillo J, González-Padilla DA, García- Rojo E, Passas-Martínez JB, Tejido - Sánchez Á. Urinary infections in patients with catheters in the upper urinary tract: Microbiological study. Urol Int. 2017;98:442–448 .

43. Gajdács M, Ábrók M, Lázár A, Burián K. Increasing relevance of Gram-positive cocci in urinary tract infections: A 10-year analysis of their prevalence and resistance trends. SciRep. 2020;10:17658 .

44. Stokes W, Parkins MD, Parfitt ECT, Ruiz JC, Mugford G, Gregson DB. Incidence and outcomes of Staphylococcus aureus bacteriuria: A population-based study. Clin Infect Dis. 2019; 69:963–969.

45. Zychlinsky Scharff A, Rousseau M, Lacerda Mariano L, Canton T, Consiglio CR, Albert ML, Fontes M, Duffy D, Ingersoll MA. Sex differences in IL-17 contribute to chronicity in male versus female urinary tract infection. JCI Insight. 2019; 5:e 122998.

46. Storme O, Tirán Saucedo J, Garcia-Mora A, Dehesa-Dávila M, Naber KG. Risk factors and predisposing conditions for urinary tract infection. Ther Adv Urol. 2019;11:17 -28.

47. López-Cruz I, Esparcia A, Madrazo M, Alberola J, Eiros JM, Artero A. Sex differences in aged 80 and over hospitalized patients with community-acquired UTI: A prospective observational study. Heliyon . 2022; 8:e 11131.

48. Kline KA, Lewis AL. Gram-Positive uropathogens , polymicrobial urinary tract infection, and the emerging microbiota of the urinary tract. Microbiol Spectr . 2016;4(10):28-32.

49. Ala- Jaakkola R, Laitila A, Ouwehand AC, Lehtoranta L. Role of D-mannose in urinary tract infections-a narrative review. Nutr J. 2022;21(18):69-102.

50. Flores-Mireles AL, Walker JN, Caparon M, Hultgren SJ. Urinary tract infections: Epidemiology, mechanisms of infection and treatment options. Nat Rev Microbiol . 2015; 13:269-284.

51. Gauzit R, Castan B, Bonnet E, Bru JP, Cohen R, Diamantis S, et al. Duration of anti-infective treatments. French SPILF and GPIPR recommendations. Journal of Pediatrics and Child Care. 2021; 34(4):175-93.

52. 1. Erba L, Furlan L, Monti A, Marsala E, Cernuschi G, Solbiati M, et al. Short vs long-course antibiotic therapy in pyelonephritis: a comparison of systematic reviews and guidelines for the SIMI choosing wisely campaign. Intern Emerg Med. 2021;16(2):313-23.

53. Fox MT, Melia MT, Same RG, Conley AT, Tamma PD. A seven-day course of TMP-SMX may be as effective as a seven-day course of ciprofloxacin for the treatment of pyelonephritis. Am J Med. 2017;130:842–5 .

54. Dinh A, Davido B, Etienne M, Bouchand F, Raynaud- Lambinet A, Aslangul -

Castier E, et al. Is 5 days of oral fluoroquinolone enough for acute uncomplicated pyelonephritis? The DTP randomized trial. Eur J Clin Microbiol Infect Dis. 2017;36:1443–8 .

55. Ahmed H, Farewell D, Jones HM, Francis NA, Paranjothy S, Butler CC. Incidence and antibiotic prescribing for clinically diagnosed urinary tract infection in older adults in UK primary care, 2004–2014. PLoS One 2018; 13:e0190521 .

56. Germanos GJ, Trautner BW, Zoorob RJ, Salemi JL, Drekonja D, Gupta K, et al. No clinical benefit to treating male urinary tract infection longer than seven days: an outpatient database study. Open Forum Infect Dis 2019;6:216-28.

57. Ahmed H, Farewell D, Francis NA, Paranjothy S, Butler CC. Impact of antibiotic treatment duration on outcomes in older men with suspected urinary tract infection: retrospective cohort study. Pharmacoepidemiol Drug Saf . 2019;28:857–66 .

58. Boel JB, Jansåker F, Hertz FB, Hartung Hansen K, Thonnings S, Frimodt -Moller N, et al. Treatment duration of pivmecillinam in men, non-pregnant and pregnant women for community-acquired urinary tract infections caused by Escherichia coli: a retrospective Danish cohort study. J Antimicrob Chemother . 2019; 74:2767–73.   .

59. Barrier . L. Urinary tract infections in the elderly: difficulties in microbiological diagnosis and impact of prescribing urine culture for the care of the elderly at Angers University Hospital. Medical thesis. Angers. Angers University, 2014.

60. Jepson RG, Williams G, Craig JC. Cranberries for preventing urinary tract infections. Cochrane Database System Rev . 2012; 10:CD001321.

61. Fongoro DA. Urinary tract infections in the elderly: epidemiological , clinical and bacteriological aspects in the nephrology department of the Point G University Hospital. [Doctoral thesis in medicine]. University of Science, Techniques and Technologies of Bamako; 2022.

62. Pickard R, Lam T, Maclennan G, et al. Antimicrobial catheters for reduction of symptomatic urinary tract infection in adults requiring short-term catheterization in hospital: a multicenter randomized controlled trial. Lancet. 2012;380(9857):1927–1935.

63. Ackermann RJ, Monroe PW. Bacteremic urinary tract infection in older people. JAGS 1996;44:927-933 .

64. Meyers BR, Sherman E, Mendelson MH, et al. Bloodstream infections in the elderly. Am J Med 1989;86:379-384 .

65. Deulofeu F, Cervello B, Capell S, Martina C, Mercade V. Predictors of mortality in patients with bacteremia: the importance of functional status. JAGS 1998;46:14-18 .

66. Leibovici L, Pitlic SD, Konisberger H, Drucker M. Bloodstream infections in patients older than eighty years. Age Aging 1993;22:431 -442.

67. Pittet D, Li N, Woolson RF, Wenzel RP. Microbiological factors influencing the outcome of nosocomial bloodstream infections: a 6-year validated, population-based model. Clin Infect Dis 1997;24:1068 -1078.

68. McGeer A, Campbell B, Emori TG, et al. Definitions of infection surveillance in long-term care facilities. Am J Infect Control. 1991;19:1–7 .

69. Pickard R, Lam T, Maclennan G. Types of urethral catheter for reducing symptomatic urinary tract infections in hospitalized adults requiring short-term catheterization : multicenter randomized controlled trial and economic evaluation of antimicrobial- and antiseptic-impregnated urethral catheters. Health Technol Assess Winch Engl. 2012;16:1-197 .

70. Lam TBL, Omar MI, Fisher E, Gillies K, MacLennan S. Types of indwelling urethral catheters for short-term catheterization in hospitalized adults. Cochrane Database Syst Rev. 2014;9:CD004013.

71. Cooper FPM, Alexander CE, Sinha S, Omar MI. Policies for replacing long-term indwelling urinary catheters in adults. Cochrane Database Syst Rev. 2016;7:CD01115.

72. Das R, Perrelli E, Towle V, Van Ness PH, Juthani -Mehta M. Antimicrobial susceptibility of bacteria isolated from urine samples obtained from nursing home residents. Infect Control Hosp Epidemiol Am. 2009;30:1116 -1119.

73. Lo E, Nicolle LE, Coffin SE, Gould C, Maragakis LL, Meddings J, et al. Strategies to prevent catheter-associated urinary tract infections in acute care hospitals: 2014 update. Infect Control Hospital Epidemiol . 2014; 35:464-479.

ANNEXES

Appendix 1: Information sheet

File No. ....

Age: .... years

Gender: M/F

Comorbidities:

− HTA: yes / no

− Diabetes: yes / no

− Coronary artery disease: yes / no

Clinical data

− Time to diagnosis (defined as the average time between the onset of symptoms and the diagnosis of UI):... ....

− Functional signs: ....

....

....

− Physical signs: ....

....

....

Biological data

− Blood count and formula (CBC):

      o GB : ....

      o PNN :... ....

      o Hg :.................... .

      o Platelets: ....

− Sedimentation rate (SSR): ....

− C-reactive protein (CRP): ....

− Blood sugar : ………………

− Creatinine: ………………

− Estimated DFG: ………………

Bacteriological diagnosis

− Blood culture: ……………………………………………………………

− Cytobacteriological examination of urine (ECBU):

- o Macroscopic appearance: clear cloudy leukocyturia

- o Microscopic hematuria: yes / no

- o Germ: ……………………………………………………

- o Antibiogram:

Antibiotics	Resistant	Intermediate	Sensitive
Penicillin			
Oxacillin			
Ampicillin			
Amoxicillin			
Amoxicillin-Clavulanic Acid			
Ticarcillin			
Ticacillin -Clavulanic acid			
Piperacillin			
Piperraciline - Tazabactam			
Cefepime			
Cefoxitin			
Cefotaxime			
Ceftriaxone			
Ceftazidime			
Cefuroxime			
Aztreonam			
moxifloxacin			
Imipenem			
Streptomycin			
Gentamicin			
Kanamycin			
Tobramycin			
Amikacin			
Netilmecillin			
Sulfamethroxasole-trimetroprim			

Chloramphenicol			
Tetracyline			
Erythromycin			
Pristinamycin			
Lincosamine			
Nalidixic Acid			
Norfloxacin			
Ofloxacin			
Ciprofloxacin			
Levofloxacin			
Vancomycin			
Teicoplanin			
Colistin			
Nitrofurantoins			
Sulfamethoxazole			
Rifampicin			
Fosfomycin			
Ertapenem			

Radiological data

– Ultrasound of the kidneys and urinary tract: ……………………………

……………………………………………………………………………………

……………………………………………………………………………………

…

– Abdominopelvic CT: ………………………………………………………

……………………………………………………………………………………

……………………………………………………………………………………

…

Therapeutic data

– Antibiotic used:

    o Molecule: …………………………………………………

    o Dosage: …………………………………………………..

    o Route of administration: ………………………………

    o Duration of treatment: …………………………………

– Interventional radiology (drainage and puncture)

– Surgery : ……………………………………………………………

Scalable data

– Evolution: Favorable or unfavorable

– Complications: ....

....

....

...

Appendix 2: Normality threshold of the biological parameters used .

Biological parameters	Normality thresholds
GB	4000 – 10000 /mm³
PNN	1500 - 7000 /mm³
Lymphocytes	1500 - 4000 /mm³
PNE	40 - 400 /mm³
GR	4 - 5.7 million/mm³
Hemoglobin	13 - 17 g/dl
VGM	80 - 95 µ³
Platelets	160,000 – 350,000 /mm³
Natremia	136 - 145 mmol /l
Kaliemia	3.5 - 5 mmol /l
CRP	< 6 mg/l
Urea	2.5 - 10 mmol /l
Creatinine	65 - 120 µmol /l

GB: white blood cells; PNN: polymorphonuclear neutrophils; PNE: polymorphonuclear eosinophils; RBC: red blood cells; MCV: mean corpuscular volume; CRP: C-reactive protein

Summary

Problematic
Urinary tract infections are the second most common reason for consultation in the elderly. They can cause systemic infection, hospitalization, sepsis and even death in frail elderly patients.

Work Goal
The objectives of our work were to study the epidemiological, clinical and paraclinical characteristics of urinary tract infection in the elderly and to detail the therapeutic management of this clinical entity.

Patients and methods
This is a descriptive retrospective study of the records of elderly patients hospitalized for a urinary tract infection in the infectious diseases department of the Hédi Chaker University Hospital in Sfax over 13 years between January 2010 and December 2022.

Results
We collected 382 cases of patients aged over 65 years who were followed for urinary tract infection with an average annual frequency of 29.4 cases/year. The average age of the patients was 75.6 ± 6.5 years with a female predominance (52.6%). Acute pyelonephritis was the most observed clinical form (84.8%). Confirmed UTIs were classified as community-acquired in 91.9% of cases and nosocomial in 8.1% of cases. Systemic inflammatory response syndrome (SIRS) was the most common sign of severity (47.4%) and 81.2% of patients were hospitalized with an average duration of 8 days . *Escherichia coli* was the most isolated germ (62.8%). For the strains of Enterobacteriaceae tested, we found a sensitivity to 3rd generation cephalosporins of 66.4% and to fluoroquinolones of 49.8%. Empiric antibiotic therapy was appropriate in 87.4% of cases. Radioguided drainage was performed in 1.8% of patients and surgical management was performed in 4.2% of patients. A favorable outcome was noted in 75.6% of patients with a mean apyrexia time of 2.1 ± 1.9 days. An unfavorable outcome was found in 21.2% of patients and mortality was 3.1%.

Conclusion
Urinary tract infection in the elderly presents distinct clinical and therapeutic particularities, requiring a personalized approach. Atypical symptoms and frequent comorbidities complicate diagnosis and treatment. Appropriate

management can reduce complications and improve the quality of life of elderly patients.

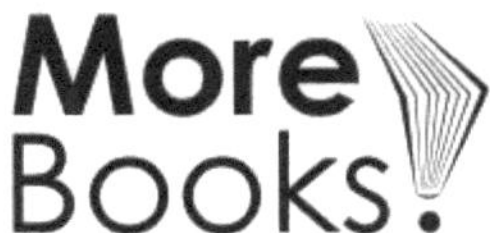

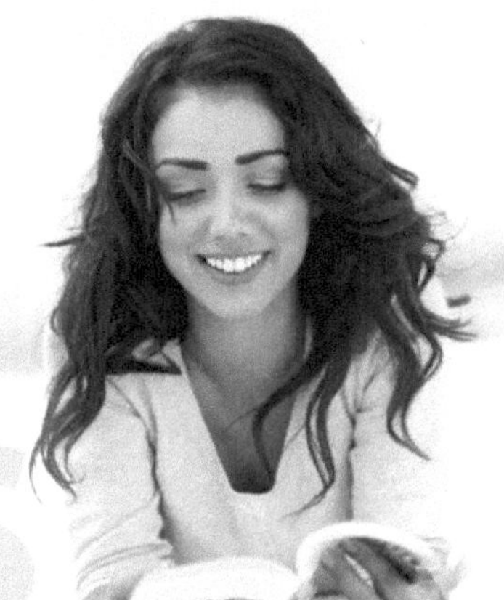

I want morebooks!

Buy your books fast and straightforward online - at one of world's fastest growing online book stores! Environmentally sound due to Print-on-Demand technologies.

Buy your books online at
www.morebooks.shop

Kaufen Sie Ihre Bücher schnell und unkompliziert online – auf einer der am schnellsten wachsenden Buchhandelsplattformen weltweit! Dank Print-On-Demand umwelt- und ressourcenschonend produzi ert.

Bücher schneller online kaufen
www.morebooks.shop

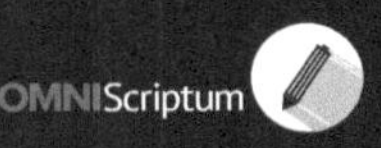